I0122620

EAT, Love GET PREGNANT

A Couple's Guide To Boosting Fertility
& Having A Healthy Baby

By Niels H. Lauersen, M.D., Ph.D
& Colette Bouchez

Ivy League Press
New York - Copenhagen - London

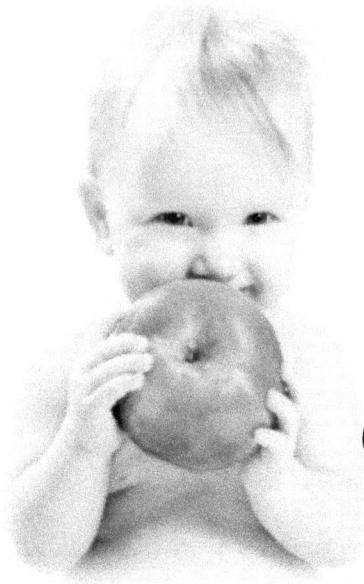

Eat
Love
Get Pregnant

To Eat …

means not just to fill your tummy with nutritious foods,
but to fill your heart and your soul with the positive
emotions that make the world a better place to be.

To Love…

means to not just love each other, but to love yourself, and
to share your love freely and unconditionally with the new
life you are about to create.

To Get Pregnant …

means to not just conceive, but to fill your hearts and your
life with the new found joy of creating a family - your
family - the most important thing there is in life.

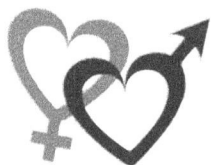

Our Dedication:

We dedicate this book to all of you now standing on the threshold of parenthood.

We ask only that you believe in yourselves, believe in your power as a couple and believe in your ability to bring into this world a beautiful, healthy, and beloved family.

We have helped thousands of couples do just that and we know we can help you too!

Niels H. Lauersen, M.D., Ph.D

& Colette Bouchez

ILP

Eat - Love - Get Pregnant: A Couples Guide
For Boosting Fertility & Having A Healthy Baby
Copyright 2010 Niels H. Lauersen & Colette Bouchez

All rights reserved. No part of this book may be reproduced or transmitted in any form or by any means, electronic or mechanical including photocopying, recording or any information storage or retrieval system without express written consent from the publisher or author. For further information contact: Info@IvyLeaguePress.com

Eat - Love - Get Pregnant may be purchased for business or promotional use or special sales. For information please
contact Info@IvyLeaguePress.com or visit www.IvyLeaguePress.com

This book is not intended as a substitute for medical advice from your physician. The reader should regularly consult with a physician in matters pertaining to her health & fertility, particularly in regard to
symptoms that may require medical attention.

The authors or Ivy League Press cannot be responsible for any results obtained or derived from information in this book. The information in this book is not considered medical advice and is offered only as a guide to getting optimal care.

Printed in the United States of America
10 9 8 7 6 5 4 3 2 1
First Edition Published 2010

ISBN: 9780615508863

Library of Congress Cataloging in Publication Data:
Eat- Love - Get Pregnant
/Niels Lauersen -Colette Bouchez

1. Conception - Popular Works
2. Reproductive Health - Popular Works
3. Natural Treatments - Popular Works

Interior and Cover Design by Elle Media
www.ElleMediaNetwork.com

BY NIELS H. LAUERSEN, MD, PhD & COLETTE BOUCHEZ

Acknowledgements

First and most importantly, we would like to thank the thousands of patients and readers of our previous books who believed in our natural health ideals. Thank you for supporting all our efforts and encouraging our continuing mission to safely and naturally help couples get pregnant and bring stronger, healthier babies into the world.

We also want to acknowledge the many medical organizations , who as we do, believe that science and nature can work hand in hand. We applaud you and we thank you for your dedication and for sharing your knowledge and research.

We would especially like to thank those organizations who so generously shared with us their expertise including The American Society of Reproductive Medicine, The American Diabetes Association, The American College of Obstetricians and Gynecologists, The Endometriosis Association, The American Botanical Society, The Journal of Complementary and Alternative Medicine, The American Association of Oriental Medicine, The National Certification Commission for Acupuncture and Oriental Medicine.

A special thank you to Poula Helth & Hans Jorn Filges for sharing with us their knowledge and expertise on the emotional side of infertility and the importance of couple communication in the quest for getting pregnant. A special thank you goes out to Linda Chard, D.C., Holistic Consultant for the NHS Fertility Clinics for your inspiration and knowledge of natural fertility therapies. To Dr. Patricia Conrad, thank you for sharing your expertise on women's health and particularly natural hormones - we are indebted for your kindness. To embryologist Carlo Acosta, your expertise is a guiding force for all couples trying to conceive.

Our deepest gratitude also goes out to our legal team and business advisors, attorney David Field, Bruce Kowal, and Albert Terranova.

And to the staff of Ivy League Press: Thank you the hard work, support and dedication . We are grateful for everything you have done to bring this book to fruition. To St. Jude: Thank you for bringing us through it again. And to Mary, for the wisdom and the love that gives us hope for the future.

EAT, Love GET PREGNANT

A Couple's Guide To Boosting Fertility & Having A Healthy Baby

By Niels H. Lauersen, M.D, Ph.D
& Colette Bouchez

TABLE OF CONTENTS

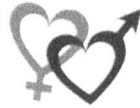

Introduction

Eat,
Love,
Get Pregnant:

A Couples Guide

Discovering you are pregnant, and giving birth to a child, are two of life's greatest joys. For a man and woman to share their love in this special and unique way doesn't just make the world go round, it makes our individual world the special place it is. To share our love not just with our partner, but with our children is, indeed, a gift that is beyond compare.

For some of you reading this book, giving and receiving this special gift will be easy. Within a few months of "trying" you will be blessed with the news that you are pregnant – bringing new joy and new meaning to your life.

For others, however, things may not go exactly as planned. For some it may simply take a little bit longer than normal to conceive – you probably know by now, that Mother Nature has her own time-table, and it's never the same for any two couples!

For still others, however, the "pregnancy timetable" may begin to extend much further than you could have imagined.   Weeks of hopefulness can turn into months of trying, and still no pregnancy occurs. And you begin to wonder … "*Could* something really be wrong – will I ever get pregnant?"

But no matter what point you are in your pregnancy journey – just starting out, trying for several months, or unsuccessful at trying for 6, 8, 10 months or more - what you will discover in this book can and will change your life.

- If you are just beginning your journey towards parenting, what you will learn in this book will not only save you time and help you conceive faster and easier, but also help insure you have a healthier baby.

- If you have been trying for a while – and getting a bit frustrated because you are not getting pregnant, this unique guide will shine the light on the simple, easy ways to identify the small lifestyle and nutritional changes that can speed up the process – and get you quickly and safely on the road to conception, and having a healthy baby.

- If you have been trying unsuccessfully to get pregnant for an extended period of time, and have grown weary and frightened that you will never conceive, this book will help you assess and evaluate your personal pregnancy obstacles and teach you how to remove them and improve your fertility– so you can conceive, and give birth to a healthy, happy, smart baby sooner than you realize.

How can I make you these promises – and be so certain they can come true? Because the guidelines featured in this book have already been tested and proven to work on thousands of couples at my own Park Avenue fertility center in New York City – and at the clinics of many of my colleagues around the world.

Certainly, if you or your partner have a serious, physiological problem standing in the way – such as blocked fallopian tube or the inability to manufacture healthy sperm – the information in this book will be extremely helpful, but it may not be quite enough to complete your journey to parenthood. For this you may need some *medical* treatment to overcome the specific *medical* problems that could be standing in your way. And the good news is that everything you will discover in this book will help maximize your fertility in ways that will encourage the success of any medical treatment you receive.

That said, I can promise that for the vast majority of you reading this book, the information you will discover - on diet, lifestyle, nutrition, natural and Chinese herbal formulas, as well as how to solve the simple medical problems that stand in the way of pregnancy – can and will make the difference between infertility and fertility. And when it comes to giving birth to your beautiful new baby, well these same suggestions will help ensure you will have the smartest, healthiest, baby possible!

How My Plan Can Help You

Throughout my 40 year career in medicine I have treated tens of thousands of patients just like you –and I have delivered more "miracle" babies than you can imagine - often to couples who believed they *never* would conceive. Indeed, with each new "miracle birth" came a new story of struggle and frustration, of anger and fear – as many of these couples tried, on their own and sometimes with other doctors to get pregnant - and just could not make it happen.

And while each patient is a unique and special individual, yet year after year I could see the success of my treatment plan – as described in this book - unfolding as one, by one, patients who could not get pregnant, or whose every pregnancy ended in miscarriage, were able to give birth to healthy, beautiful babies.

As time went on and new research appeared, I was pleased to see that the natural approach which I had personally studied and developed for all these years was also being proven over and over in clinical studies. Moreover, as new research began to appear, providing even more evidence on the power of natural treatments to encourage pregnancy, I began to incorporate these new findings into my treatment plan as well . The end result was a program that could help even more couples to conceive - even when they were told by other doctors there was no hope.

Finally, earlier this year, I decided to make this successful program available to everyone – and the idea of *Eat, Love, Get Pregnant* was born. I chose this title because

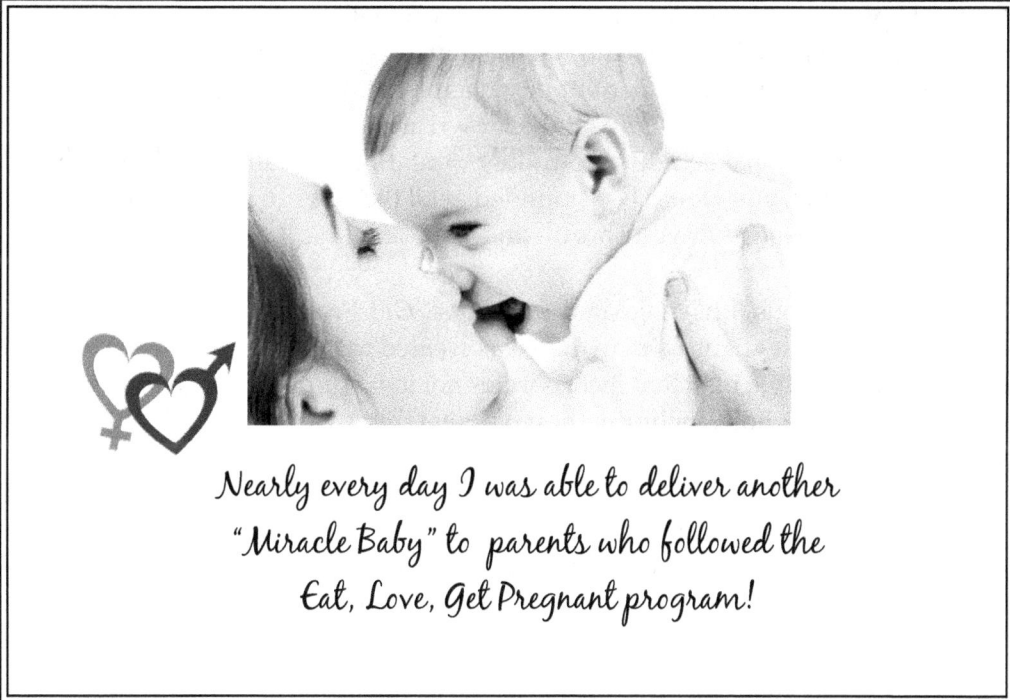

Nearly every day I was able to deliver another "Miracle Baby" to parents who followed the Eat, Love, Get Pregnant program!

of the simple, yet powerful nature of this plan – a program that is so easy to follow, yet so effective that it will benefit every couple planning to conceive.

A Breakthrough Couples Guide To Getting Pregnant

But as proud and as happy as I am to bring you not just the latest research, but the proven aspects of a program that has already helped thousands of couples conceive, I wanted to add still something more to this book – something I found was lacking in nearly all fertility and pregnancy books. And that is, the importance of couples working together, as a team, supporting one another and deepening their bonds of intimacy - and the important role that this too can play in a successful conception.

Indeed, what many couples can never realize is that in the course of trying to find the road to parenthood, they detour off the path that led them to each other to begin with. I have seen many loving, soul-mate relationships all but crumble under the weight of trying to have a baby.

But perhaps more important was the recognition that when a couple works together, within the bonds of love and intimacy towards a common goal, they can have a powerful impact on each other's body chemistry. In fact, it can be an impact so strong that it has the ability to affect their own and their partner's fertility in myriad ways. From hormonal activity controlling ovulation to brain chemistry controlling sperm production, you would be astounded at all the ways in which your relationship affects so many aspects of your health and your fertility.

For all these reasons, I have created *Eat, Love, Get Pregnant* to be a true "couples" guide to getting pregnant – a plan that was created to be read and shared by the both of you. It is a lifestyle plan that incorporates not just your individual bodies, but your relationship as a whole, including how you eat, how you play, and how you share your love.

Certainly you will find sections of this book that apply just to male fertility or female fertility, with specific suggestions according to gender. But what you will also find, as a theme running throughout this book is the importance of your relationship and your love, as it pertains to getting pregnant.

For this reason it is my hope that not only will you and your partner read this book together, but that *Eat, Love, Get Pregnant* will help strengthen the bonds between you – and help you to always remember the real reason you wanted to have a baby to begin with: To show your love for one another by creating another wonderful human being to complete your life together.

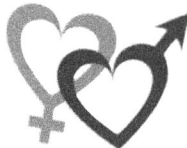

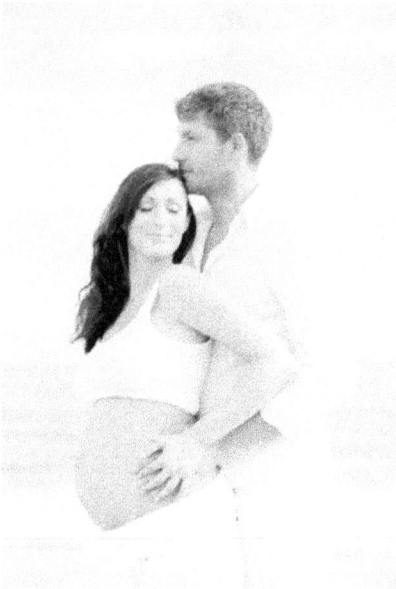

Chapter One

Understanding Your Fertility:

What Every Couple Needs To Know!

When it comes to getting pregnant I am a firm believer that lifestyle – including diet, nutrition, and stress control - can be your biggest assets, or your greatest downfall. Indeed, most couples never realize just how big a role their lifestyle plays in every aspect of their health – including their fertility.

And so, as this book unfolds, chapter-by-chapter you will learn not just the ways in which your lifestyle can affect your fertility, but how to harness the power of simple lifestyle changes to give your fertility a super boost. Not only will the secrets in this book help you and your partner maximize your physical health in ways that will have a positive impact on your fertility, but they will also have a direct and immediate impact on many aspects of your reproductive health and on the steps it takes to conceive quickly and have a healthy baby.

But before you and your partner begin that journey, it's important that you both take a few minutes out to learn a little bit about the "natural science" of getting pregnant - including how sperm and egg meet and what happens when they do!

It is my hope that having this basic understanding will not only allow you to make more use – and more sense – of what you read in the remainder of this book, but also allow you to use these suggestions in a way that will most benefit you and your partner's specific fertility profile.

So without further ado, let us begin your journey to parenthood with some important basic information on just how your fertility functions and how together you and your partner can work as a team to create a brand new life.

Life Begins With Hormones ...

If you've ever suffered a bout of PMS, or even if you've just felt cranky and bloated a few days every month, then you have already experienced the power of three important reproductive hormones: Estrogen, progesterone and testosterone.

But it's not just your body that is affected by these chemicals - your partner is as well. Indeed, he has the *same three hormones* coursing through his body as well - but in much different amounts.

For example, while you have lots of estrogen (the egg-producing hormone), some progesterone and a very little bit of testosterone in *your body* , your partner has the opposite equation. He has lots of testosterone (the sperm-making hormone) , and very little estrogen and progesterone.

Another key difference: While you experience fluctuations in the levels of these hormones during every monthly menstrual cycle – in your partner levels remain constant. Why is this difference so important?

Because hormone levels remain constant in men, it means that sperm is continually being produced every single day. This means that anytime a man is intimate with a woman he has the potential to create a baby.

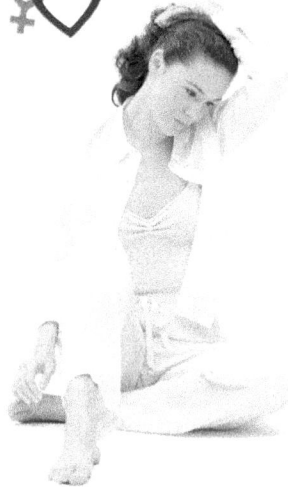

Unlike a man whose hormones remain constant, a woman's hormones continually fluctuate - which is one reason why women suffer with PMS and men do not!

But it's actually these fluctuations that tell you that you are fertile and that you can get pregnant!

Women, on the other hand, have a completely different type of reproductive system at work – one that is in fact rooted in these hormonal fluctuations. Certainly, you may not always be happy about the way those fluctuations sometimes make you feel – they are, in fact, the reason why women experience PMS and men do not – but the fact that these biochemical ups and downs *do occur* is really your fertility blessing in disguise. Because the truth is, without the movement of estrogen and progesterone, conception could never occur!

How The Brain Helps A Woman Get Pregnant

As important as your key reproductive hormones are, leading the way for these important fluctuations to occur in women is a series of natural biochemical events - all steps, by the way, that are necessary to get pregnant. The goal of all this natural biochemical activity is to not only stimulate and control the fluctuation of estrogen and progesterone, but in the process help your egg develop, grow and be released from your ovary in a process known as ovulation. In fact, only after this occurs can your egg meet up with your partner's sperm to make pregnancy happen.

While some of these important bio-chemicals are made in your ovaries, some of the key ones are actually produced and released by your brain. Or, at least stimulated by the release of brain chemical signals. In fact, your brain is really where the whole process of getting pregnant actually begins!

The most important of these brain chemical signals include the following compounds:

1. **Follicle Stimulating Hormone or FSH** - Secreted by the pituitary, a tiny gland located inside your brain, the job of FSH is to send a signal to your ovaries to produce an egg. While every woman is born with a lifetime supply of egg follicles (the estimate is that there are about 400,000 follicles inside your ovaries from the time you are born) without stimulation from FSH, they would never mature into an egg.

2. **Luteinizing Hormone or LH -** Also secreted by your pituitary gland, this hormone instructs your matured egg to leave the ovary in the process known as ovulation, and directs it to travel down the fallopian tube where it can meet with your partner's sperm allowing fertilization to occur.

Together these two hormones are known as "gonadotropins". While there is some FSH and LH in your body at all times, these levels fluctuate. Moreover a significant amount is released during the first half of your menstrual cycle – when your egg is maturing, developing, and getting ready to be ovulated. This is followed by a dropping off of both hormones after ovulation. To help orchestrate the timing of this rise and fall is a third hormone. It's known as:

3. **Gonadotropin Releasing Hormone or GRH.** Secreted by the hypothalamus (a tiny gland located in your brain just above the pituitary gland) the job of GRH is to direct the release of the proper amounts of FSH and LH into your bloodstream at *the proper time.*

Together the function of all of these hormones is to orchestrate the rise and fall of your two main reproductive hormones directly involved in making eggs and helping those eggs to become fertilized, implant and eventually grow into a baby. These key hormones are:

4. **Estrogen** - Manufactured primarily inside your ovaries, levels rise and fall as result of a direct signal from the brain hormone FSH, which in turn helps orchestrate egg production. A surge in estrogen around the time of ovulation also provides more vaginal lubrication which in turn can increase your desire for sex, and help your partner's sperm travel more easily through your vagina and cervix. And both of these things help encourage conception.

5. **Progesterone** – Manufactured by the corpus luteum - the shell that your ovulated egg leaves behind - the job of this hormone is to work with estrogen to help prepare your uterus to receive a fertilized egg, *and* help it to be nourished and grow.

How Your Body Prepares You For Conception

Now that you are familiar with key hormones involved in getting pregnant, it's important to know something about how they all work together! Indeed, like the finely tuned harmonies of a great musical group, your entire network of reproductive hormones work together to set the stage for conception to occur.

The entire process goes something like this:

- At the start of each monthly menstrual cycle, your GRH messengers sense that your estrogen levels are low – a sign that you are not pregnant. This in turn sends a signal to your pituitary gland to step up in the production of FSH, which is necessary to stimulate both estrogen and ultimately, egg production.

- As FSH production increases, many follicles inside your ovary begin to develop. As days pass, however, usually only one pulls ahead of the rest in growth and development.

Eventually it becomes your "egg of the month" – the one that will be released and become available for fertilization. At the same time the growth of this egg causes your ovaries to produce more estrogen, and the level rises quite quickly and dramatically. This serves two purposes. First, it helps your egg to mature to the point where it *can* be fertilized. And second, it works with progesterone to stimulate the lining of your uterus to thicken, so that in the event your egg is fertilized, there will be a thick, spongy "nest" to receive it! But equally important, when estrogen levels rise and reach a specific point, it sends a signal to your brain that your egg is ready

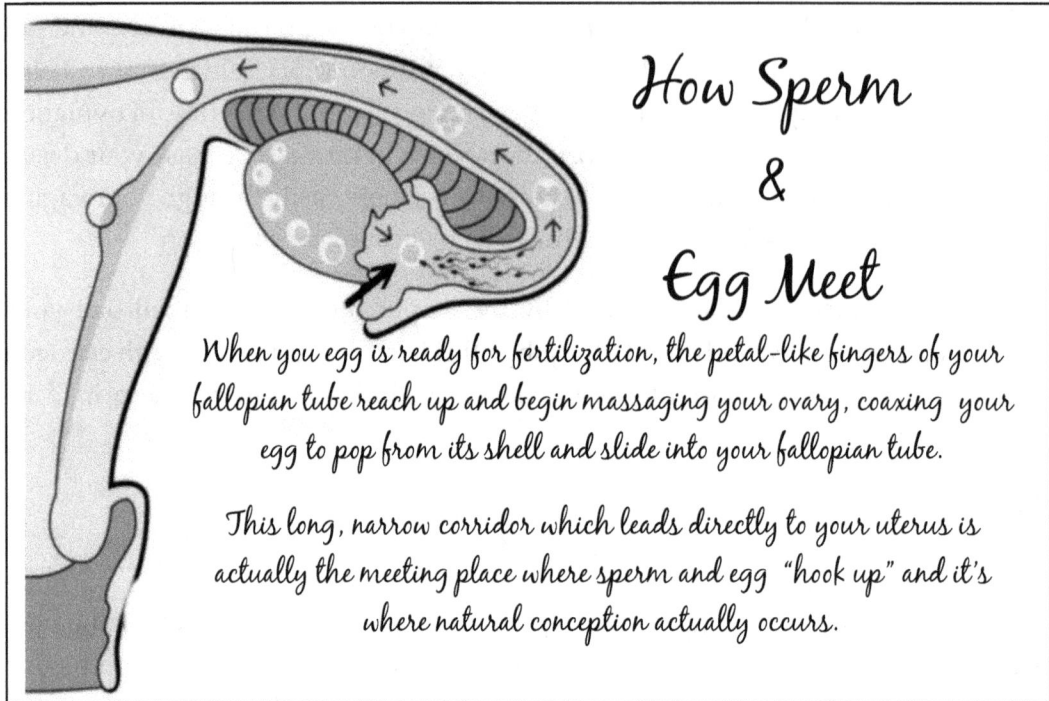

How Sperm & Egg Meet

When you egg is ready for fertilization, the petal-like fingers of your fallopian tube reach up and begin massaging your ovary, coaxing your egg to pop from its shell and slide into your fallopian tube.

This long, narrow corridor which leads directly to your uterus is actually the meeting place where sperm and egg "hook up" and it's where natural conception actually occurs.

to be released. This in turn causes the release of the brain hormone LH – which as you remember is the what prompts your "ripe and ready" egg to pop from your ovary in a the process known as *ovulation*.

This is key, since it is only after ovulation occurs that your egg can meet up with your partner's sperm so that fertilization can take place. In fact, failure to ovulate is one of the key reasons many women have problems getting pregnant.

The Final Step: Introducing Egg To Sperm!

While this finely tuned biochemical and hormonal network is intrinsic to getting pregnant, none of this would matter if your egg could not hook up with your partner's sperm. And while it may seem this is just a matter of *chance*, the truth is, the "set up" is very much intentional! There is, in fact, a purpose- driven introductory process that occurs between sperm and egg – think of it like the beginning of your relationship with your partner, where, step by step, one date at a time, you eventually fell in love!

Indeed, the preparation for the big "sperm and egg date" actually begins the moment your egg begins to mature and gets ready for ovulation. When it does, petal-like fingers that sit at the far end of your fallopian tube reach up and begin massaging your ovary, creating a kind of gentle suction that works to coax your egg to pop from its shell and slide into the portion of the fallopian tube connected to your ovary.

This long, narrow corridor which leads directly to your uterus is actually the meeting place where sperm and egg "hook up" – and it's where natural conception actually occurs. This is one reason why the health of your fallopian tubes is so intrinsic to getting pregnant – they provide the actual environment for sperm and egg to get together, and the healthier and problem -free that environment is, the easier it will be for egg and sperm to unite. A little later on you'll learn some important natural ways to encourage a better fallopian tube environment so that egg and sperm have the optimum conditions under which to meet.

But getting back to that egg-sperm 'date' – what can also help increase the chances that a connection is made is directly related to the activity of your partner's sperm, millions of which are being produced every single day. In fact, unlike a your body, which produces just a single egg every month, your partner's body is busy churning out sperm 24/7, every single day. Indeed, every time your partner ejaculates into your body, he is releasing thousands of sperm, all of which compete to be "the one" to fertilize your egg.

But while there may be thousands of sperm available for conception, it's important that they begin making their journey into your body at the right time – just before, or just as , your egg is being released. And this is where the concept of ' "good timing" plays a key role in getting pregnant. How and why does this work?

Once your egg has ovulated, it remains fresh enough to be fertilized for just 24 hours or less. This means if your partner's sperm does not "hook up" with your egg in that time frame, the chance for pregnancy dramatically declines. In fact, one of the key mistakes couples make when trying to get pregnant is waiting until ovulation to begin making love. If you do this, then there is barely enough time for your partner's sperm to meet up with your egg before it begins to disintegrate and the window of conception opportunity is lost . Or if conception does occur at this late stage, often the resulting embryo can be "defective", which often results in a miscarriage.

On the other hand, because sperm can live in a woman's body for up to 5 days – and still be fresh enough to fertilize an egg - making love 3 to 5 days prior to when you are expected to ovulate will help insure your partner's sperm are ready and waiting for your egg the moment it arrives! And this dramatically increases your chance for a quick and healthy conception! (Later in this book you'll learn some key ways to know when you are going to ovulate, and predict the day and time up to 5 days in advance!)

But even assuming you do make love at the right time – beginning before ovulation occurs - you may be wondering how sperm knows exactly *where to go* to find your egg. The "mating call" so to speak, begins with your cervical mucus, which opens channels that allows the sperm to move forward through your uterus to your fallopian tubes.

But one of the more interesting newer discoveries made about the "egg-sperm" mating dance was the recognition that inside the head of each sperm is a sort of biochemical "radar" that literally picks up a signal being silently emitted from a developing egg . This natural "come hither" signal actually tells sperm where to go, and pulls it to the egg. I like to think of this as a kind of "silent" mating song that helps naturally draw sperm and egg together the same way two soul mates are destined to meet.

What's interesting to note, however, is that as complicated as this may sound, the whole process can take place rather quickly . Studies have shown that when a man is healthy and strong, eats well and gets the proper nutrients, he makes sperm that are healthy and strong enough to swim from the vagina to the fallopian tubes in as little as ten minutes.

Once this meeting of sperm and egg does occur there is, however, still one more biochemical process that must take place before conception can happen. Namely, one of partner's many sperm must penetrate and enter your egg – a step that allows your DNA to combine with his DNA and begin to form your baby. To make this happen, all available sperm immediately attach to the outer shell of your egg. This process initiates still another chemical step – this one causing the release of a substance located in the head of the sperm that is designed to break down the outside shell of the egg allowing entry.

Although all the sperm are competing for the chance to be "the one" that gets inside, much like your mate who worked to win your heart, generally one sperm works a little harder and a little faster than all the rest, enabling the entry process to begin.

Although all the sperm are competing for the chance to be "the one" that gets inside, much like your mate who worked to win your heart, generally one sperm works a little harder and a little faster than all the rest, enabling the entry process to begin.

Once this occurs, much like supportive teammates on the football field, the other sperm stop their "drilling" process and pull away from the egg – thus giving the "lead sperm" a chance to gain entry. (The other sperm, by the way, swim away from your egg and within a few days die off and are bio-chemically dissolved by fluids in your body).

Once the strongest sperm gains entry into your egg, the fertilization process begins inside your fallopian tube. After sperm and egg combine an embryo is formed and the cells begin to divide - first into two cells, then four, then eight. While this is happening, the cilia, which are tiny hairs that line the inside your fallopian tube, begin slowing moving your developing embryo towards your uterus - which by the way is another reason it's important to keep the environment of your tubes healthy and open.

With this distinct sense of natural timing in play, your embryo should reach your uterus or "womb" at approximately the 8 cell stage (about 3 days after fertilization) – the time when it is easiest for your baby to attach to the newly thickened lining of your uterus so it can be nourished by your body and begin to grow and develop.

To ensure that this nourishment phase continues – not only now, but throughout your pregnancy - both estrogen and progesterone levels remain high. This in turn signals your brain to keep FSH and LH production at a minimum – which also prevents any new egg follicles from being stimulated into growth and development. This is why your menstrual cycle stops and you can't get pregnant during this time.

If, however, for any number of reasons fertilization does not occur, levels of both estrogen and progesterone drop rapidly. It is this rapid drop in hormone levels that causes the spongy lining inside your uterus to break down and be shed. This shedding process becomes the basis of your menstrual bleed.

Once that bleeding stops – within about 7 days – your body is once again ready to start a new cycle wherein you once again prepare to grow and release a new egg, and another chance for conception occurs.

When Pregnancy Doesn't Happen: What Goes Wrong

If you're like many of my patients, you may be wondering why making love at the 'right time" doesn't automatically lead to pregnancy *every time* – and why it can take so long to get pregnant.

First, it's important to remember that no matter how much medical science has learned about conception there is still some indefinable "magic" involved!

Sometimes, even when all conditions are right for pregnancy – a healthy egg is made and ovulated at the right time, and a hearty group of healthy sperm is ready and waiting to pounce – still conception might not happen. It's this indefinable impact of Mother Nature that ultimately reminds those of us in the science world who is really in charge!

But that said, there are also a number of biological, even medical reasons why conception does not occur each and every time you have intercourse – *even at the right time of the month.*

The first and easiest explanation is that not every woman ovulates every single month. While regular ovulation is more likely when you are in your teens and early twenties, you may be surprised to learn that by your mid to late twenties, ovulation can be a bit irregular. This is particularly true if, like most women you have a full, multi-tasking life, a less than optimal diet, and your life is filled with stressed.

And one of the key secrets you will discover in this book is not only how your diet can help encourage a more regular ovulation, but also how to use specific stress reduction techniques and small changes in other lifestyle factors to encourage more frequent and regular ovulation.

These same factors, by the way, can also influence how sperm behaves, so even if you are ovulating regularly, your partner may not be producing a ready supply of mature, healthy sperm – or the sperm that are produced may not be "energetic" enough to swim upstream and reach your egg.

Some can even lose their way entirely, and never even reach your fallopian tube. And this is where simple changes in diet and lifestyle can make a huge difference in helping your partner produce more, better, more energetic and heartier sperm, which will also encourage conception odds.

For some couples, however, there can sometimes be a bit more serious problems getting in the way the way of conception - some of them so silent you might not even know they exist – until you try to get pregnant.

Factors That Impact A Woman's Fertility

1. **Blocked fallopian tubes -** This can result from a biological problem such as endometriosis (a menstrual related disorder – see below) or a sexually transmitted infection that may have been contracted many years before and lived "silently" in your body . This is often the case with Chlamydia, one of the leading sexually transmitted infections linked to fertility problems. Moreover, infections and endometriosis can each lead to the formation of "adhesions" or scar tissue, which form blockages that trap sperm or egg, prevent an egg from entering the tube, or block sperm and egg from meeting. If the scarring is not too severe, laser surgery can remove the blockages and free the tubal pathways, so getting pregnant can be much easier.

2. **Ovarian malfunction** - This can mean a reduced ability of your ovary to produce a healthy egg, or the inability of that egg to leave your ovary during ovulation. This can be the result of a hormonal snafu, or, commonly related

to a condition such as PCOS – poly cystic ovary syndrome. In this condition the ovaries fail to function normally, so eggs are not readily produced or released. Often this is treatable with medication and diet (see Chapter 12).

3. **Uterine Blockage –** This can include problems with the shape or size of the uterus itself , or, as is much more often the case, the result of fibroid tumors , polyps, or scar tissue or adhesions resulting from previous surgery, all of them inside the uterus and capable of interfering with implantation. Most often fertility-sparing treatment involves removal of the fibroids or polyps, and/or treatment with medication, which in turn can help restore your fertility so you can get pregnant .

4. **Endometriosis:** This is a menstrual related disorder that causes an over-growth of uterine tissue either within the uterus itself, or in other areas of the reproductive system, including the fallopian tubes or ovaries.

   This excess tissue can form blockages or create adhesions in any of these organs, block ovulation as well as create a hormonal imbalance that interferes with fertility. Endometriosis can be treated with medication or surgery, as well as with diet and lifestyle changes. (See Chapter 12 for a more thorough look at this common condition and how it affects fertility.)

5. **Hormonal Deficiency –** This is a wide sweeping problem that can include everything from a metabolic malfunction – such as thyroid disorder that alters the production of FSH and LH - to an ovarian problem that curtails the production of estrogen or progesterone, or impacts the amount or consistency of your cervical mucus.

   It can also be caused by an over production of other hormones – including the stress hormone cortisol – that in turn can impact the production or timing of all the hormonal steps essential to conception.

   The bottom line: You may not produce eggs, or the eggs you produce may not be ovulated or released, or the lining of your uterus may not be thick and spongy enough to properly nourish an embryo.

In all cases diet and lifestyle changes, and sometimes hormonal therapy, can make a huge difference when it comes to getting your reproductive life back on track. You can also read more about each of these problems in much greater depth, as well as the treatments for these problems, in my book *"Getting Pregnant: What You Need To Know."*

Turning Back The Hands of Time

Science has known known for quite some time that as a woman ages, she makes fewer, and lesser quality eggs . And we also know that this can translate into a reduced chance for getting pregnant - beginning at around age 35.

Now however, we also know that age affects men and sperm production as well. In fact, as a man ages, he experiences not just a reduction in the amount and quality of the sperm he produces, but also a reduction in the ability of that sperm to successfully navigate through a a woman's body and locate, and ultimately fertilize, her egg.

So while age may impact your fertility faster, and at a more dramatic rate than it impacts your partner, he is by no means immune to age-related effects on fertility.

What Interferes With A Man's Fertility:

- Blockages or infections in the epididymous (the area of a man's reproductive system where sperm are made).

- Blockages within the vas deferens, (the area where sperm mature, grow and are released).

- Problems within the system which helps transport sperm from his body, into his penis, and ultimately into your reproductive system.

Moreover, many men are not even aware a problem exists since oftentimes there are no obvious outward signs that something is wrong.

The good news however is that in nearly all instances, seeking treatment with a urologist (a male fertility specialist) will dramatically improve a man's sperm profile, regardless of any problems that might exist.

The Good News: You Will Get Pregnant!

As complicated –or even discouraging - as all of this may sound, there is good news to report as well. As many opportunities as there are for things to go wrong while trying to get pregnant, there are equally as many opportunities for you to take control and make them go right! And one of the key ways to do this is via the diet and lifestyle changes you will find throughout this book. Not only will they help set the stage for a faster, easier, healthier conception, but at the same time improve your health in ways that will offer you myriad benefits – many of which can also help turn even the most devastating fertility odds around.

Other important factors you will also read about in this book – such as the impact of stress reduction on fertility as well as the fertility benefits of cultivating and keeping a loving, warm relationship with your partner - will also help you get pregnant faster and easier as well.

Of course there is no one "magic bullet" or "magic change" that does everything. Instead, all of the small changes work together in harmony to bring about the big changes in your fertility.

Remember, a healthy body is a fertile body – so when you do good things for your body and your overall health, your fertility benefits as well!

At the same, I would be remiss if I did not mention that, for a small percentage of you reading this book, a physiologic barrier to pregnancy could exist – one that will require a medical intervention to "level the playing field" and correct the underlying physiological roadblocks to conception. And, indeed, if you have been trying to get pregnant for more than 12 months, or if you are over 35 and have been trying for over 6 months, it's probably a good idea to see a fertility specialist and have some basic tests to see if there is a problem that might require treatment. If this turns out to be true, the earlier you seek treatment, the easier it will be to get pregnant.

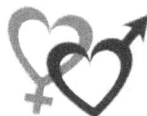

Chapter Two

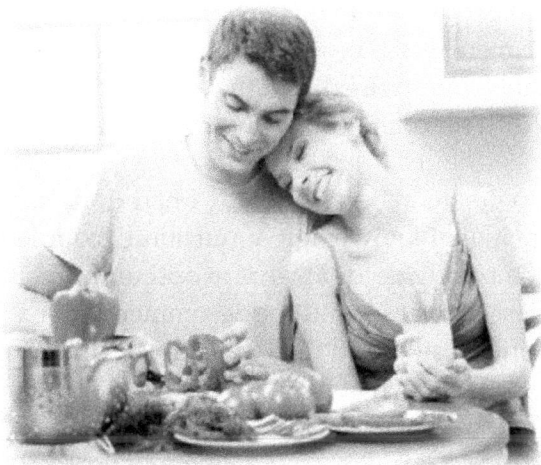

Eat Smart
&
Get Pregnant
Easier

How Food Can Boost Your Fertility!

It's hard to open a magazine or go online without seeing a story about diet. Indeed, it sometimes seems that everywhere we look food is playing an increasingly important role in our health and our lives. And I'm not just talking about weight control!

Indeed, over the past decade and especially these last few years there has been an amazing amount of research showing that what we eat – as well as what we avoid eating – can have an enormous impact on helping us not just avoid disease, but in some instances even reverse it. And nowhere is this adage more true than when it comes to fertility.

Today we have the research to prove what I and so many of my European colleagues have believed in and lectured about for decades: Diet and fertility go together like peanut butter and jelly - with certain foods, *and some specific food combinations*, having an almost uncanny power to bring about baby making success. Sometimes they can be so powerful they help turn a couple from infertile to fertile in just a matter of months.

Indeed, having grown up in Denmark, in a family that was very aware of the power of healthy eating, I learned early on the importance of good nutrition. Having received both my undergraduate and medical school education in the capitols of Europe – where diet has always remained a health priority – my feelings about the importance of good nutrition continued to capture and hold my attention. When, in the 1970's I came to America to practice medicine , I brought with me not only the idea that diet and fertility were unmistakably intertwined, but that by tweaking the diets of my patients I could help make a difference in how easily they conceived.

And so, long before it was fashionable to create a "fertility diet", I had done so – based not just on research, but on my personal knowledge of nutrition, coupled with my own intuitive feelings about what the body needs to work at optimum levels. I am proud to say that many of my earliest theories – and the recommendations I made to patients for many years - not only resulted in many healthy and happy pregnancies, but have also been proven via research at many of the world's most prestigious universities. From Harvard, Yale, Columbia and Stamford in the United States, to the top medical schools in France, Germany and England, scores of researchers have worked hard to bring us more and more proof that when it comes to getting pregnant, your diet can play a major role.

But it's also important to realize that it's not just female fertility that is affected by diet - male fertility is affected as well. Indeed, while your baby will be conceived, develop and grow inside *your body,* one half of the success of your pregnancy, and your baby's health, is dependent on your partner's sperm – the health of which can and often is directly related to what he eats. As such, it's not just your pre-conception diet that matters, but your partner's diet that makes a difference as well.

So whether you are just thinking about getting pregnant, or if you and your partner have had difficulty conceiving or suffered miscarriages, I am happy to tell you that, as a couple, making small but simple changes in what you eat can make a huge difference in helping your parenting dreams come true.

The Foods That Boost Fertility:
What To Eat Right Now

Today, nearly all couples are aware of the need to eat healthier during pregnancy. For example, most pregnant women know the importance of including foods rich in the nutrient folic acid in their diet – which helps prevent a group of serious birth defects.

But in truth, it wasn't really until the 1980's that we had proof this was so! Indeed, the links between a healthy pregnancy and a healthy diet are much more recent than people realize.

In much the same way, it wasn't until the last several years that we began to see not just the importance of eating right *during pregnancy*, but also the role that diet can play during the pre-conception period as well. We now know, for example that if a woman is short on certain important nutrients while she is trying to conceive, she may not ovulate regularly, or the eggs she does create may not be healthy enough to be fertilized.

Likewise, men who come up short on certain key nutrients may see the results in sperm that are slow to move, are weak or cannot swim straight, and often too few in number to fertilize an egg!

The flip side of this food coin: We also have strong proof showing that both men and women who take the extra steps to fortify their fertility through a healthy diet not only get pregnant faster and easier, but also have healthier babies. While food certainly can't fix every reproductive problem, it can and does play a major role in maximizing your fertility .

So, whether you are trying on your own to conceive, or you're already working with a fertility doctor, paying attention to what you eat, and eating the right combinations of foods, can bring you that much closer to realizing your parenting dreams!

What *should* you and your partner eat to maximize your fertility and encourage pregnancy? The first stop on the fertility food train is at the Farmer's Market – where you'll find the very fertility foods that your Mom told you to eat more of from time you were a child: Fruits and Vegetables.

Mother Knew Best!

The very same foods that Mom encouraged you to eat when you were young - fruits & vegetables - can also act as powerful fertility foods for you and your partner when you are trying to conceive!

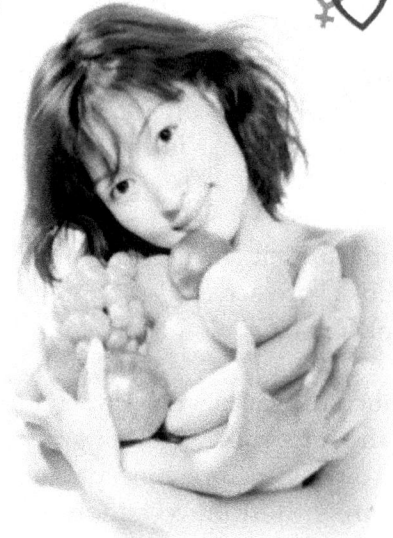

Fruits, Vegetables and Conception

Over the past decade, and particularly during the last several years research concerning the health benefits of fruits and vegetables has been nothing short of astounding. Proving once again that Mom was definitely right when she cautioned us to "Eat all your vegetables or no dessert" , the health benefits of all sorts of produce can no longer be denied.

From adding much-needed fiber to our diet, to providing us with the vitamins and nutrients we need to help fight heart disease, diabetes, even cancer, the benefits of eating 5 fruits and veggies every day is now considered one of the best preventive health measures men and women can take.

But apart from the fertility benefits that come from simply having a healthy body, we also have discovered that fruits and vegetables, particularly some specific types of produce, can have some direct effects on a number of key factors involved in the process of making a baby. From impacting the hormones involved in healthy egg production and eventually ovulation in women, to influencing factors involved in the sperm manufacturing process in men, to helping overcome a somewhat illusive group of problems known collectively as "unexplained infertility", we now now that fruits and vegetables will make a huge difference in many areas of your reproductive health.

But how and why does this happen – and which fruits and vegetables are likely to do you the most good? It all starts with understanding a few basics about good nutrition – and how these factors are intimately entwined with your fertility.

And that understanding begins by exploring a series of natural compounds known as "phyto-nutrients" - naturally occurring chemicals that are present in some specific fruits and vegetables, and are now believed to play an intrinsic role in not just helping the body maximize good health, but also improve your fertility profile.

While virtually all produce has health value, providing a good source of both fiber and a variety of nutrients important to overall health, when it comes to your fertility it is, in fact, the fruits and vegetables highest in "phyto nutrients" that play the most important role in helping you get pregnant.

By learning more about what these compounds are, how they work, and where to find them, you can begin to create your personalized fertility food plan – a diet that will help you and your partner boost your overall reproductive health and even help combat some specific fertility challenges.

PhytoNutrients and Getting Pregnant:
The Secret Fertility Foods!

One of the unique things about the plants that yield our fruits and vegetables is that they don't possess the same kind of natural "warning" system about impending dangers that both humans and animals have . For example, I'm sure you're familiar with the adrenalin fueled " fight or flight" response – that natural surge of hormonal activity that occurs when we are in danger, giving us the strength to "fight or flee" our attackers. And while it may seem that the ability to do this is a product of modern living, the truth is, these natural biochemical responses were programmed into our DNA millions of years ago.

Protect Your Fertility With Phyto-Nutrients!

Phyto-nutrients can become the protective umbrella that prevents both your egg and your partner's sperm from damage caused by exposure to environmental factors - factors that might otherwise harm the DNA, which is the genetic material necessary to conceive a healthy baby!

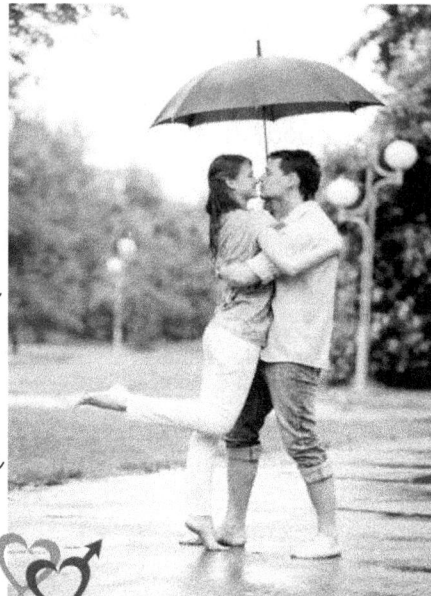

Unfortunately, however, plants don't possess this same "fight or flight" chemical process. But fear not – because Mother Nature provided something equally as effective – a natural chemical warning system that protects them from danger.

This system is a natural chemical network known as "phytonutrients". In fact, in the plant world, the sole purpose of phytonutrients is protection from assault – be it from insects, a fungus, or even many of the very same environmental threats that can harm you, including the damaging rays of ultra violet light from the sun. And herein lies one of the keys as to how phytonutrients can protect you as well.

By tapping into this same powerful natural network of protection, phytonutrients can give your body some distinct advantages, including helping to counter the effects of cellular damage that occurs from not just exposure to environmental toxins such cigarette smoke and air pollution, but also the effects of stress and the impact of a diet loaded with junk food, too much alcohol, and not enough "healthy" foods.

The Power of Phytonutrients – And Why They Work

For a great many years, researchers believed that the health benefits of eating fruits and vegetables came solely from their vitamin content – specifically the "antioxidant vitamins" such as C, E and beta carotene. And in fact these nutrients are still important – and you'll learn why in just a little while.

But over the past decade, and particularly in the last five years, researchers have uncovered an even greater benefit to eating these foods. And that is the benefits provided by phytonutrients – factors which researchers now believe are even more important to good health than the vitamins and minerals these foods also provide.

Indeed, in one very interesting study researchers actually caused intentional damage to a strand of DNA – the basic genetic compound that forms the basis of all life. They then treated that broken strand of DNA with different types of phytonutrients as well as with vitamin C. Using a computer to analyze the results they found the combination of phytonutrients did a better job at repairing the DNA than the vitamin C alone.

But how does this relate to your fertility? Every time your body experiences an environmental, dietary or lifestyle assault, there is the potential to damage the DNA necessary to create healthy eggs, and allow these eggs to be fertilized. By tapping into the powerful, natural protection that phytonutrients provide, you can prevent at least some of that DNA damage from occurring. It may even help to repair damage that has already occurred. Either way, the end result is a natural boost to your fertility.

But it's not just women –or eggs – which are affected in this way. Interestingly, the impact of phytochemicals on DNA was also echoed in a study on sperm. In research published in the journal *Teratogenisis, Carcinogensis and Mutagenisis* researchers found that certain phytonutrient compounds were able to help sperm damaged by environmental factors, thus increasing the ability to fertilize an egg.

So what should you and your partner be eating to gain the benefits of phytonutrients? Certainly, a well rounded diet containing lots of different fruits and vegetables can go a long way in ensuring your nutrient intake. However, in terms of optimizing your fertility, there are several key phytonutrients that play an especially important role in conception .

Choosing foods highest in these nutrients *can* give an extra boost to your fertility and help reduce the rate of many personal biochemical snafus that could be standing in the way of getting pregnant. Moreover, by incorporating these foods into your pre-conception diet you will not only improve your chances of conceiving, but when you do get pregnant you'll be giving your baby the very best and most nutritious start to life.

What To Eat To Get Pregnant

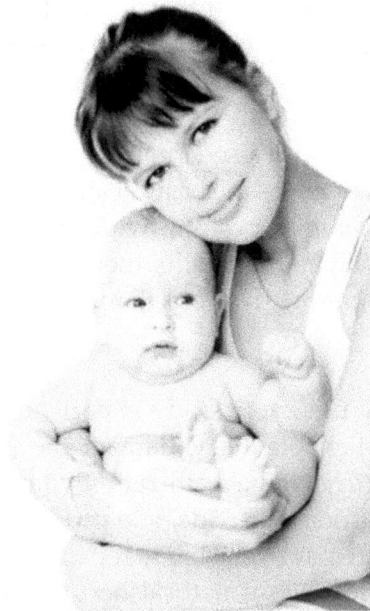

While there are literally thousands of phytonutrients found in fruits, vegetables, nuts and grains – and all of them good for your health - when it comes to boosting fertility, the most important ones can be grouped into just three categories. They are: *Phenolic acids, flavonoids,* and *carotinoids.* While each group contains a number of individual phytonutrients, their power really comes from working together as a team.

In fact, I'm quite certain that at least some of the foods found in these individual groups – such as green tea – are items you've already heard about in terms of fertility boosting powers. But again, the real "power boost" comes not from isolating one or two foods from each of these groups, but in creating meals that utilize phytonutrients from all three groups, which, when eaten together work as team to do your fertility the most good.

Moreover, you will notice that some fruits and veggies fall into more than one "phyto-nutrient" group – meaning they contain more than one set of nutrient compounds. So, whenever possible, choosing these "double duty" foods will give you an even bigger bang for your nutrient buck! So what should you eat to put the "team" to work? What follows is an easy-to-use guide to the most important phytonutrients and the foods that contain them!

By eating foods deep and rich in color - particularly the color red - you will ensure your body is getting a good supply of phenolic acid - the natural compound that protects your reproductive health from environmental toxins like cigarette smoke and air pollution.

Fertility Phytonutrient Group # 1 : Phenolic Acids

Phenolic acid – also known as "polyphenols" - are compounds that help protect the body from pollutants, repair damage caused by cigarette smoke and air pollution, and offer protection from heart disease.

One particular type of phenolic acid making huge headlines right now is "reservatrol". It's actually manufactured by plants in response to environmental stress, so, it's not hard to see why it is so closely associated with overcoming the effects of oxidative stress on cells.

Foods high in this compound can not only protect your heart, but your blood vessels - key to ensuring good blood flow to your ovaries and your uterus. But they have also been shown to protect the overall health of every cell involved in conception!

To increase your intake of polyphenols eat more:
- Red or purple fruits such as grapes, raspberries, strawberries, pomegranates and cranberries.
- Citrus fruits but particularly red grapefruit.
- Wine made from red grapes.
- Walnuts and pecans.

Fertility Phytonutrient Group # 2 : Flavonoids

This group of nutrients has a direct impact on blood pressure, plus they support the heart and aid capillaries in maintaining good circulation, all of which is key to healthy egg production and ovulation.

A type of flavonoid known as quercertin (found in grapes as well as in cherries) helps keep tiny particles found in blood from sticking together and forming clots, which may help some women reduce their risk of miscarriage.

Another flavonoid known as catechins – found in green tea - pack a heavy punch against cancers of the reproductive system, as well as heart disease.

But it is really the impact of two more specific flavonoids - compounds known as anthocyanin and proanthocyanidin - that may help your fertility the most. Why? They work to reduce the production of "cytokines". These are inflammatory compounds produced by various cells in the body that can impact fertility. Indeed, studies show that inflammatory compounds can exert subtle but important negative effects on everything from egg production , to ovulation and egg transport.

Inflammatory compounds can even create such a hostile environment for sperm that they don't want to swim anywhere near your egg – and some simply perish and die before they even get through your reproductive system!

Moreover, since fat cells are one of the major producers of cytokines, if you carry even a few extra pounds on your frame, then you are automatically over-producing cytokines.

In fact, it is the overproduction of inflammatory cytokines produced by fat cells that many believe is one of the reasons that women who are overweight generally have a harder time getting pregnant.

In addition, these same inflammatory compounds can also play a role in insulin resistance and PCOS, as well as endometriosis – all conditions that impact fertility.

But the good news is that by including foods high in flavonoids in your diet, and by specifically choosing foods high in the compounds anthocyanin and proanthocyanidins, you can counter at least some of the negative inflammation while at the same time optimizing your fertility.

Beverages like green or black tea, fruits such as peaches or grapes and vegetables like lentils or black eyed peas are loaded with flavonoids – natural chemicals that protect the reproductive system.

To increase your intake of flavonoids eat more:

- Tea , and particularly green tea which contains 3 times the flavonoid content of black tea, plus it also contains a flavoinoid known as catechins which has protective effects on the entire reproductive system. In addition, grapes, cocoa, lentils, black eyed peas, peaches and nectarines are also good general sources of flavonoids.

- You can increase your intake of quercertin by eating more red grapes, cherries, kale, lettuce, apples, pears, nectarines, peaches, broccoli and onions, as well as drinking more tea.

- Gain the fertility-boosting effects of anthocyanin and proanthocyanidins by adding more blue-red fruits to your diet including blueberries, raspberries, strawberries, loganberries, cherries, currants, pomegranates, grapes and cranberries.

Fertility Nutrient Group # 3: Carotinoids

The best known in this powerful group of nutrients is the compound beta –carotene. As you probably already know this is the nutrient your body uses to help manufacture vitamin A, which is a key key fertility nutrient, essential to the healthy growth and development of your embryo. In fact when a serious vitamin A deficiency exists it's almost impossible to create a healthy embryo – so it becomes impossible for a pregnancy to thrive and survive.

But as important as beta carotene is, when it works together with other carotinoids – such as lycopene and lutein - the power to impact your entire reproductive system is astounding. Indeed, research published by the *European Society of Human Reproduction and Embryology* demonstrated how a number of compounds within the carotinoid family are essential to healthy follicular fluid – the semi-liquid substance which surrounds your egg and aids in growth and fertilization. Because follicular fluid appears to get its supply of beta carotene from the bloodstream, it stands to reason that when levels are low, eggs may not fertilize as easily.

Equally important, animal studies have shown that beta carotene impacts the release of LH – luteinizing hormone, the brain chemical which signals the release of your egg and actually allows ovulation to occur.

Moreover, a healthy corpus luteum (the shell your ovulated egg leaves behind) is naturally rich in beta carotene. Since this is the major source of progesterone, the hormone that helps prepare your uterus for a healthy conception, fortifying it with additional beta carotene helps to optimize hormone production necessary for a healthy implantation.

When it comes to increasing sperm health, one particular member of the carotinoid family – a compound known as "lycopene" - has been shown to be especially important. Moreover, without an adequate supply of all the carotinoids (they actually make up 1/3 of the content of each sperm), levels of LH and subsequently testosterone can drop so low that sperm can no longer be made!

So it's easy to see why,when levels of this nutrient are low, sperm production can falter. This can result in not just a low sperm count, but in a greater percentage of defective sperm - making a healthy fertilization much more difficult to attain.

Tomatoes, watermelon and carrots are three foods high in carotinoids and they are especially good for both male & female fertility.

So be sure you and your partner share these delicious treats together, and often!

To increase your intake of carotinoids eat:

- Carrots, butternut squash, tomatoes, sweet potatoes, cantaloupe, kale and mangoes- all of which contain most of the full complement of carotinoid compounds.

- To specifically add more lycopene to your diet eat more tomatoes, watermelon, guava, plus red and white grapefruit.

- To maximize levels of lutein eat more avocados, oranges, and leafy green vegetables.

- For even more beta carotene try apricots, papayas, plantains, broccoli, celery, pumpkin, spinach and winter squash.

Super Food Protection: The Anti Oxidant Connection

As you have just read, there are clearly some specific fruits and vegetables that can make a huge difference in your fertility. And it's important that you try to include at least 5 of the fruits and vegetables chosen from the three groups I just mentioned.

But that said, I don't want you to think that the other fruits and vegetables which are not on this list are not important – *because they are*. In fact, almost every fruit and vegetable on the planet offers at least one or more specific health benefits. But when it comes to getting pregnant perhaps the greatest advantage of this food group as a whole, is the ability to protect you from what are known as "free radicals".

This is a type of renegade cell that can do *enormous* damage to your body and specifically to your reproductive system. But what are free radicals , and how can they harm your fertility?

Essentially, free radicals are a type of malformed oxygen molecule that is missing one of its components. Normally, healthy oxygen molecules – which are found throughout our body - contain an inseparable pair of tiny particles called "electrons." Think of them as a loving couple who wants to be together all the time!

In the case of free radical oxygen molecules, however, one of those electrons is missing. And so, the lonely free radical molecule is always on the hunt, trying to find it's electron mate. And while this may sound like a sad biochemical "romance novel", the truth is, the lonely free radical in a ruthless hunter – a kind of tiny molecular "assassin " which roams through your body targeting any healthy cell it can find and tries to disable it, thus stealing the missing electron.

The worst part of this: The process by which the free radical tries to get inside the healthy cell - which involves a chemical conversion known as "lipid oxidation". This activity generates the production of still more free radicals, which in turn are set loose in your body looking for still more cells to destroy.

But what causes free radicals to begin with – and how do they affect your fertility?

First, it's important to know that the creation of free radicals is part of our natural body chemistry. They are made in response to the to the aging process of cells – a process, which you may be surprised to learn begins the moment you are born and continues throughout your lifetime!

But it's not these free radicals you have to worry about. Because if you are in relative good health, the body naturally quenches *these* free radicals soon after they are generated – and long before they can attack healthy cells and do any real harm.

Unfortunately, however, that's not always the case with free radicals generated by a number of environmental and lifestyle factors - including a diet high in saturated fat and animal fat, exposure to tobacco smoke (including second hand smoke), exposure to chemical toxins from pesticides or even household chemicals, and especially overexposure to the burning rays of the sun. All of these factors can cause your body to produce more free radicals – far more than what is produced naturally.

So what does all this have to do with your fertility – and your ability to get pregnant? Once a free radical gets inside a healthy cell, it begins to immediately attack and alter the factors necessary for healthy cell function - including damaging the DNA, the very essence of each cell's life function.

When enough DNA damage to enough cells occurs, it paves the way for not only a number of diseases to set in – including cancer, diabetes, Alzheimer's, and Parkinson's – but also impacts fertility in myriad ways.

Indeed, dozens of studies now show that in one form or another free radicals – and their resulting oxidative stress cell damage - can impair fertility by:

- Impacting the ability of your eggs to mature and develop.

- Interfering with your ability to ovulate on a regular basis.

- Causing or exacerbating changes in the lining of your uterus, making it difficult for your embryo to attach and grow.

- Impacting the lining of your fallopian tubes, keeping your fertilized egg from reaching your uterus.

- Creating a hormonal imbalance significant enough to interfere with fertility on many levels.

Indeed, one study published in the *Journal of Human Reproduction* in 2007 suggested free radical cell damage occurring in a woman's body can have such a direct impact on conception, it could completely block her ability to conceive.

In another study published in the same journal in 2008 doctors found that when the follicular fluid surrounding a woman's eggs was exposed to the kind of oxidative chemical stress released by free radicals, those eggs not only became damaged, but as such, were much less likely to be fertilized.

Explaining Unexplained Infertility: The Free Radical Connection

Anytime a couple has problem getting pregnant it has the potential to become a source of frustration, anxiety, even anger. But perhaps the most devastating of all diagnosis is one of "unexplained infertility" – meaning that doctors know something is wrong, but they can't pinpoint the exact problem or the cause, or the treatment necessary to allow pregnancy to occur.

According to the American Society for Reproductive Medicine, some 50% of all couples who seek help from a fertility expert come away with this very diagnosis. Since many more couples do not seek medical help for their fertility problems, I and many other doctors estimate the number of couples affected by "unexplained infertility" is much greater than we know.

But while doctors may not know the exact cause of unexplained infertility, we do know what can contribute to the problem. And for many couples it is free radical damage – a problem that effects not just women and egg production and release, but men as well.

Indeed, research now shows that male fertility, and the production of healthy sperm is also impacted by free radical damage, thus increasing the risk of male fertility problems.

Moreover if, as a woman, you suffer from fertility robbing conditions such as endometriosis or PCOS, the additional cell damage that occurs from free radical exposure can exacerbate your condition, thereby making conception that much harder to achieve.

But what is most important for you know is that while both free radicals and the resulting oxidative cell stress can have an enormous impact on your fertility, you have the power to change your body chemistry! And while it made seem hard to believe, all you need do to take control of your fertility, is make a few small changes in y o u r daily diet.

What To Eat To Protect Your Fertility From Harm

As you may have already guessed, when it comes to protection from free radical damage, there is, perhaps, no greater warrior willing to come to your defense than fruits and vegetables. How do they help?

First, they are brimming with natural compounds known as antioxidants – vitamins like C, D, E and beta carotene. Much like the name implies, these "antioxidant" vitamins are loaded with molecules designed to prevent "oxidative damage" from occurring . How does it work?

 Once ingested, antioxidants literally float through your body searching for and "scavenging" out free radical molecules When they find them, they surround the molecule, latch on tight and work their way inside. This disarms and disables the original free radical, resulting in a much weaker new molecule that is much less able to attack healthy cells. They also work to help prevent new free radical molecules from forming.

Moreover, antioxidants also work to protect the normal healthy cells in the body, in part by reinforcing their outer membrane, making it much harder for free radicals to get inside and cause the kind of damage that can disrupt your fertility.

Lastly, in a situation where more is definitely better, fruits and veggies also help encourage your body to produce more of its own supply of antioxidant compounds, including lipoic acid. And this in turn helps to squash even more free radical production , and more importantly dramatically reduce free radical cell damage.

So, with fewer free radicals able to cause damage, and fewer free radicals being made overall, it paves the way for your good health – and your fertility – to thrive ! And this, in fact, is exactly what a number of studies have found.

But what's also key is that antioxidants work together in kind of "protection network" that creates a chain reaction of events that eventually stops the ability of free radicals to harm healthy cells. For example vitamin E disarms a free radical, but in the process produces a vitamin E radical – which then requires Vitamin C to disarm. The same is true for many other antioxidants , all of which work together in a harmonizing balance to keep the level of free radicals from getting out of control.

This is just one reason why eating foods high in only one vitamin or one type of antioxidant won't give you nearly as much protection as eating a balanced diet high in a number of different antioxidants. This balance is not only important to maintaining your fertility but also in protecting your overall health.

In research published in the *Journal of Human Reproduction* in 2008, findings suggest that a diet high in many antioxidants can favorably influence not only how quickly and easily an egg can be fertilized, but also whether or not the resulting embryo will survive and thrive – or be lost to an early stage miscarriage.

And I can tell you from my personal patient population that many women who were referred to me because of *repeated* miscarriages were able to stop the cycle of loss and give birth to a healthy baby, simply by adding more antioxidant-rich foods to their diet.

But it's not just protection against pregnancy loss that foods high in antioxidants can accomplish. Indeed these powerful nutrients also have the ability to neutralize a host of fertility-robbing factors - and in the process not only increase your ability to get pregnant right now, but also protect your fertility well into the future. So, you can continue to get pregnant – and add to your family - at your own pace.

In fact, when combined with the power of phytonutrients, fruits and vegetables also high in antioxidants offer one of the best natural fertility defense plans available! Not only can they protect you from damaging influences that can keep you from getting pregnant, they can also keep your body chemistry humming along in a way that helps ensure all of your reproductive hormones remain at the level necessary to bring about a fast , and most importantly, a healthy pregnancy.

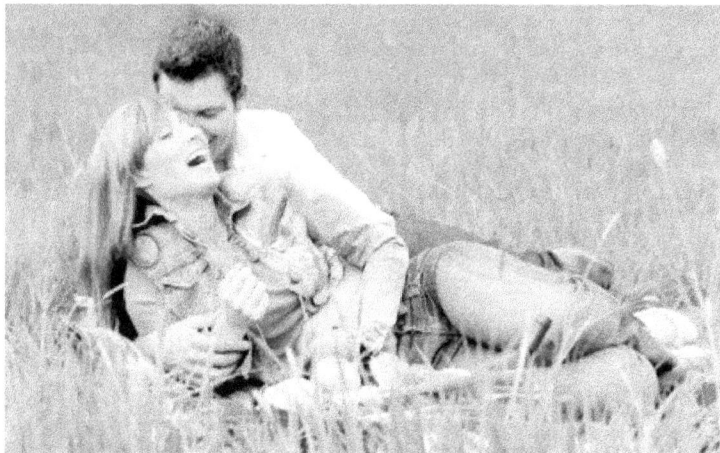

Sharing a picnic lunch that includes fruits like blueberries, cranberries, blackberries, plums and pecans can ensure that you protect your fertility while getting closer to your partner!

The Top Twenty Foods For Antioxidant Protection

To help define the foods highest in antioxidants, scientists at the United States Department of Agriculture (USDA) developed a rating system known as the "ORAC Score".

This stands for Oxygen Radical Absorbance Capacity – or more simply put, the ability of a food to absorb free radicals and keep them from causing harm.

While many foods contain relatively high levels of antioxidants, some contain a whopping amount – so much so that you only need a few servings a week to reach the recommended 3,000 ORAC units a daily needed to maintain good health.

Based on the ORAC scores, turn the page to find a listing of the top 20 foods highest in antioxidants, ranked in the order of how much they contain. The list also contains their ORAC score per serving. As you will see you don't need to eat a lot to get this valuable antioxidant protection so, Bon Appetit!

ORAC Score Top 20 List of Fertility Foods

1. Red Beans - 13, 727 ORAC units per ½ cup serving.

2. Wild Blueberries – 13, 427 ORAC units per 1 cup

3. Red Kidney Beans – 13, 259 ORAC units per half cup

4. Pinto Beans – 11, 864 ORAC units per half cut serving.

5. Regular Blueberries – 9, 019 ORAC units per 1 cup

6. Cranberries – 8,983 ORAC units per 1 cut serving.

7. Artichoke Hearts – 7,904 ORAC units per 1 cup

8. Blackberries – 7,701 ORAC units per 1 cup serving

9. Prunes – 7,291 ORAC units per ½ cup serving.

10. Raspberries – 6,058 ORAC units per cup

11. Strawberries – 5,938 ORAC units per cup

12. Red Delicious Apple – 5,900 ORAC units per apple.

13. Granny Smith Apple – 5, 381 ORAC units per apple.

14. Pecans – 5, 095 ORAC units per 1 ounce.

15. Sweet Cherries – 4,873 ORAC units per cup

16. Black Plums – 4, 844 ORAC units per plum

17. Russet Potato (Cooked) 4649 ORAC units per potato

18. Black Beans – 4181 ORAC units per half cup

19. Plum (light color) – 4118 ORAC units per fruit

20. Gala Apple – 3,903 ORAC units per fruit.

Six Super Fertility Foods: What Helps Most

In addition to the powerful fruits and vegetables already mentioned , I have what I call my list of "secret fertility weapons" - super fertility foods that have been shown in medical studies to have an enormous impact on reproductive health.

Though fruits and vegetables are certainly on my list, so are some key nuts, seeds and grains, all shown in studies to have significant nutritional impact on fertility.

On a personal note I'd like to add that I have often recommended these foods to my patients, with excellent results. Not only have these foods improved their overall health but I could see measurable results in how they also impacted their fertility, in many instances becoming the turning point that took them from infertile to fertile. As such, I urge you and your partner to include these foods in your weekly – and if possible - your daily diet. I know they can make an important difference for you as well!

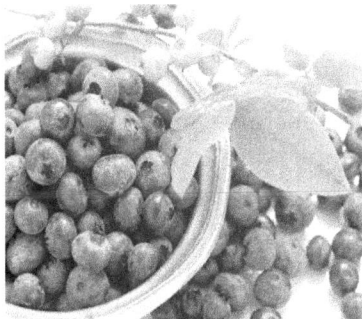

Super Fertility Food#1: Wild Blueberries

In addition to being one of the foods highest in antioxidant protection, these tiny fruits are also packed with a powerful phytonutrient known *anthocyanin* – a natural compound that is actually responsible for giving this fruit it's rich color.

As you read earlier, this important nutrient is a powerhouse when it comes to boosting fertility, as it helps reduce the impact of inflammation body-wide. This not only insures that you will make and ovulate healthier eggs, but by reducing inflammation in your fallopian tubes it clears the path for sperm and egg to meet.

And this means your embryo has a better chance of making it to your uterus at the right time, so a healthy implantation can occur. And because these same phytonutrients help keep the lining of your uterus healthy, this fruit will also dramatically reduce your risk of miscarriage.

My Recommendation: ½ cup of wild blueberries daily up to 5 days a week.

Super Fertility Food #2: Cruciferous Vegetables

Fill your plate with broccoli, cauliflower, Brussels sprouts, kale , cabbage and bok choy and you'll be giving your fertility the royal treatment! An interrelated group of produce known as "cruciferous vegetables" these green, crunchy veggies are packed with phytochemicals, as well as vitamins, minerals, and fiber that can provide you with a powerful antioxidant punch!

In one study funded by the National Cancer Institute, researchers found that body-wide oxidative cell stress (including that which adversely impacts fertility) dropped by 22% after just a few weeks of a diet high in cruciferous vegetables. Now if you think you can get the same effects by popping a vitamin supplement, guess again. The study also showed that those who took a vitamin supplement *instead* of eating their veggies saw nowhere near the same level of decrease in oxidative stress.

In addition, studies have shown that these same veggies also promote healthy estrogen metabolism and they do so through two compounds known as I3C and DIM. How do these natural chemicals affect estrogen?

There are two pathways through which you metabolize the estrogen your body produces. One pathway results in an essentially healthy metabolic byproduct known as 2-hydroxyestrone, a type of estrogen that encourages fertility. The other pathway results in the production of a more toxic by-product, a chemical known as 16 alphahyroxyesterone – which is not helpful to fertility .

In fact, a number of studies have now reported that women who metabolize estrogen into this compound are more susceptible to breast cancer. Other research indicates fertility may also be affected.

Now, here comes the vegetable link: The compounds I 3C and DIM appear to help shift the way estrogen is metabolized in your body, encouraging you to produce more of the healthy estrogenic metabolites and produce less of the more toxic type.

While studies show that this can reduce your link to both breast and cervical cancer, I, and many of my colleagues believe that encouraging the production of healthy estrogen while decreasing the production of unhealthy estrogen can also impact fertility in a positive way.

While research in this area is still new, I have personally seen the important difference that adding these vegetables to the diet can make for my own fertility patients.

Indeed, this powerful estrogenic effect, in consort with the high antioxidant potential of these same foods means you are giving your fertility a double shot of encouragement that can help maximize your chances for getting pregnant.

My Recommendation: Three to four ½ cup servings of cruciferous vegetables a day will offer you optimal protection. That said, it's important to note that eating even just one to two servings per day can also have enormous benefits. The highest nutrient values can be achieved if you choose fresh veggies and eat them raw or lightly steamed. But, you can also gain benefits from frozen or even canned veggies, you will just need to eat a bit more to reach the optimal nutrient levels. And remember, you can see a difference in as little as three weeks!

Super Fertility Food # 3: Onions and Garlic

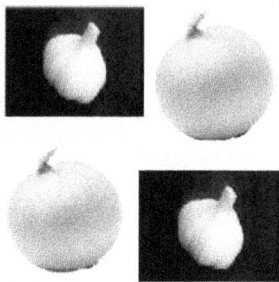

Both these vegetables belong to the family of phytonutrients known as "allyl sulfur compounds" - a group that also includes leeks, scallions and chives, and other "bulb" vegetables.

But it is onions and garlic that alone, or especially together, that pack the biggest punch in terms of protecting your health and your fertility. How can they help?

In terms of your overall health, studies show that compounds found in these vegetables are potent anti-cancer fighters - helping to protect against colon, stomach, breast and in particular ovarian cancer. In fact, studies show adding these vegetables to the diet even *after* cancer has been diagnosed, can help slow the growth of some types of malignant tumors.

In terms of your fertility, these foods can also play a key role in helping to repair damage to DNA, as well as regulating the life cycle of a cell. Indeed, one of the ways in which fertility can become impaired is via exposure to environmental toxins and pollutants – factors which ultimately break down cell walls and alter DNA. Thus, it stands to reason that any natural compounds which can halt this process can't help but boost your fertility.

But the protection doesn't stop here. In a study published in the *Journal of Nutrition* in 2003, researchers found that extracts made from garlic powder also had a potent effect on levels of cytokines – the inflammatory chemicals that, as you read earlier, can impact fertility on many levels, particularly in those women diagnosed with either endometriosis or Poly Cystic Ovarian Syndrome (see Chapter 12).

Moreover, garlic is a potent source of the mineral selenium, which is key to sperm production in men. So making sure you and your partner get your share of onion and garlic is one way you can both insure your fertility.

My Recommendation: Use onions and garlic as a garnish or in salads, at least a few times a week. To help neutralize breath odors: Toss in a sprig or two of parsley or watercress.

Super Fertility Food #4: Green Tea

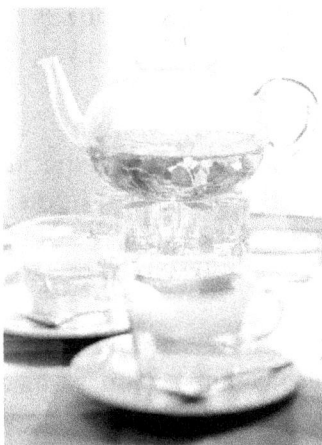

As I mentioned to you a little earlier, all teas are a wonderful source of the phytonutrient known as polyphenols – a type of flavonoid with robust antioxidant activity! While these same polyphenols are also found in black tea, the amount in green is about 3 times greater, giving you a more potent source of protection against damaging free radicals.

A second chemical that is plentiful in green tea – a natural compound known as hypoxanthine – is the same compound found in the follicular fluid that surrounds your egg in your ovary and helps to foster it's growth and development. As such, a number of researchers now theorize that drinking green tea may have beneficial effects on egg production and growth. Indeed, in one now-classic study published nearly a decade ago, researchers from Kaiser Permanente Health System found that women who drank as little as one-half cup of caffeinated green tea daily nearly doubled their chances of conceiving!

The same effect was not seen with other caffeinated beverages.

More recently, a Stanford University study of 30 women, aged 24 to 46 who had not been able to conceive for up to 3 years found that a supplement containing green tea and several other herbs and vitamins improved conception odds considerably.

Indeed, one-third of the women taking the supplement were able to conceive within 5 months, compared to no pregnancies in the placebo group.

What we don't know however, is whether or not green tea alone would have had the same effect.

That said, if the findings of a new European animal study translate to humans, green tea may indeed, be the catalyst that increases fertility.

In research published in April 2008, researchers from the University of Bologna reported that when used in conjunction with IVF , a compound found in green tea known as EGCG increased pregnancy rates significantly, mostly by increasing the number of eggs available for fertilization.

Interestingly, however, when concentrations of EGCG were increased too high, the percentage of eggs produced actually went down. So, while a little may be good for fertility, too much could be bad!

While there are no *specific* studies on the impact of green tea on *male fertility*, certainly the powerful antioxidant content can have beneficial effects on sperm production, reducing the amount of abnormal sperm while increasing the amount of normal sperm available for fertilization.

And this can only increase your chances for conception.

As with most factors that impact your health, however, moderation is the key! While it seems clear green tea can have beneficial effects on fertility, overdoing may not be a good thing.

My Recommendation: Up to 7 cups of green a week is likely to benefit you and your partner in terms of both your overall health and your fertility. But until we have more information I would limit it to that amount.

Super Fertility Food # 5: Almonds, Walnuts, Cashews and more!

Although foods that are high in fat are generally not good for your health, this tenet changes dramatically when it comes to nuts.

Indeed, there are almost 300 different types of nuts , and while they are high in fat (and calories) it's the type of fat they contain that makes them a healthy choice – and even a super fertility food. How can they help you?

First, nuts contain mostly monounsaturated and polyunsaturated oils. These are the "good fats" that can help lower cholesterol and have anti-inflammatory effects on your cells. (You'll read more about the power of good fats in the next chapter.)

But equally important, most nuts also contain a good amount of healthy omega 3 fatty acids, which as you will discover a little later in this book, helps strengthen cell membranes and protect against fertility-robbing free radical attacks.

In addition, nuts, as well as many types of seeds are also high in a natural compound known as "phytosterols" - a type of plant based fat that recently gained lots of attention for its ability to lower cholesterol.

But these healthy "sterols" do much more than that! Studies show they also work to boost your immune system – and therein may lie a secret connection to boosting your fertility as well. How? In now classic research conducted at Mt. Sinai Medical Center by my colleague, fertility expert Dr. Norbert Gleicher it was discovered that women who were prone to fertility problems had a significantly higher level of autoimmune antibodies- natural chemicals that occur as a result of malfunctions within the immune system.

Not only did these women have higher levels of these antibodies in their blood, but also in the fluid surrounding their fertilized egg.

In one study of women with abnormal levels of autoimmune antibodies who underwent IVF, Dr. Gleicher found pregnancy rates were only 1/5th of those women who had normal blood levels of these same antibodies.

So, doing what you can to keep your immune system strong will not only help protect your overall health, but could also have a direct impact on the health of your egg, *and your ability to get pregnant.* And eating nuts is one easy way to get the protection you need.

Also important to remember: Nuts are very high in protein, which , as you will learn later on in this book, is another key to healthy ovulation and egg production. But unlike meat and other animal sources which can be loaded with saturated fats, the protein found in nuts is healthier overall.

Lastly, because nuts are a potent source of fiber, they help balance blood sugar, and reduce the risk of insulin resistance, which in turn may help keep ovulation on track for some women.

In terms of your partner, nuts can also be a fertility booster since many varieties contain high concentrations of both selenium and vitamin E, two very important nutrients necessary to ensure regular production of healthy sperm. So, it's also important that you keep a bowl of nuts around the house so that you can both grab a handful now and then!

Nuts: The Best Ones For Boosting Fertility

What kind of nuts are best for fertility? It's a good idea to vary the type of nuts you eat, since each variety contains a slightly different nutrient compound.

But if you love almonds, well you are in luck! Not only do they contain the healthy fats I mentioned earlier, they are also one of the richest sources of antioxidants!

According to researchers from Tufts University, after testing the skins and kernels of 8 varieties of California almonds , they found the phytonutrients contained in these nuts offered the highest level of free radical damage protection of any flavonoid group!

In fact, what many people do not realize is that, ounce for ounce you're getting the same level of phytonutrient protection in nuts that is found in broccoli, black and green tea, and red onions! And it's a snack food!

Of course nuts can also be high in calories – so you don't want to overdo it! A hand full of mixed nuts a day is plenty to give your fertility a boost!

Plus, if you eat them instead of a typical "junk food " snack – like some chips or cookies – you'll keep your calorie intake balanced and do a good deed for your body and your fertility !

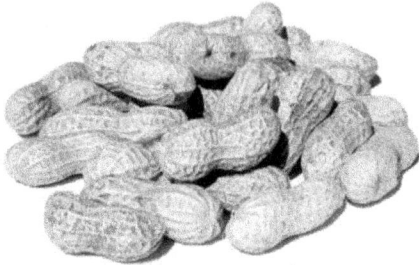

A Nutty Caution

Although all nuts have health benefits, the one type you should try to limit – and your partner should definitely *avoid* while you are trying to conceive -is peanuts. Why?

Peanuts are high in a natural compound known as "isoflavones" which is a significant source of plant estrogens. If you have an estrogen deficiency – or if you are past age 35, a time when estrogen levels naturally begin to dwindle – then eating peanuts could be helpful to you .

But, if you are young and your estrogen levels are normal, or as is often the case, above normal in relation to the hormone progesterone (one tell-tale sign is raging PMS before every menstrual cycle) then the estrogens found in isoflavones might tip your fertility balance in the *wrong direction.*

While eating a small handful of nuts a day probably won't " rock your estrogen boat", if you do find that eating peanuts increases your symptoms of PMS, then it might be affecting your fertility as well, in which case you should eat less.

In terms of your partner, it is , in fact, the plant estrogens found in peanuts that could be harmful to sperm production. This impact is doubled if he munches on peanuts while drinking beer or red wine, both of which can also act as a source of certain plant estrogens. Indeed, studies show that if the intake of these plant estrogens is high enough, it could overpower testosterone production, causing sperm count to plummet.

The latest studies from the Medical Research Council in Cambridge, England revealed that plant estrogens found in both beer and peanuts can have a clear detrimental effect on sperm and in the process make getting pregnant more difficult. So at least while you are actively trying to conceive, it's a good idea if your partner avoids beer, red wine and peanuts.

My Recommendation: A handful of mixed nuts every other day for you and your partner, eliminating peanuts for him, and for you if there is any chance your estrogen levels are too high.

Super Fertility Super Food # 6:
Pumpkin, Sunflower Seeds, & Wheat Germ

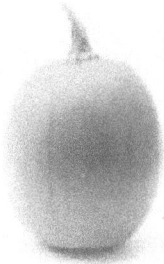

While we don't often think of foods such as sunflower or pumpkin seeds as a typical fertility food – they certainly can be!

In fact, together with wheat germ – the "embryo" or inside of a kernel of wheat – they can pack a powerful punch on not just your health, but also your ability to conceive. How? First they are powerful plant sterols, which as you just read can impact your immunity and ultimately your fertility.

But they also contain fairly high concentrations of omega 3 fatty acids – which, as you will learn a little later in this book, can boost fertility in a variety of ways, including stimulating production of sex hormones in both men and women.

Because pumpkin seeds are high in vitamin E and zinc, they can be particularly beneficial for male fertility. Research shows that just ¼ to ½ cup a day can boost the overall health of a man's reproductive system and increase the concentration of healthier sperm in each ejaculation.

If you are prone to miscarriage – or just want to ensure an extra healthy implantation - be sure to add more wheat germ to diet. High in both vitamin E and selenium these are two nutrients are essential for ensuring a healthy implantation and reducing the risk of miscarriage.

Wheat germ, along with sunflower and sesame seeds are all high in vitamin B6, which is essential to the production of female hormones and in maintaining the proper ratio of estrogen and progesterone necessary for conception.

My Recommendation: One-quarter to half-cup of either pumpkin or sunflower seeds for you and your partner; a sprinkling of wheat germ on cereal or in stews or sauces several times weekly.

Chapter Three

The Foods For Fertility Success:

Comfort Carbs, Healthy Fats & Tasty Proteins

There is perhaps nothing that can make one feel quite as good as a plate filled with what I like to call "comfort foods" - dishes like mac & cheese, a juicy cheeseburger, pasta and meatballs, or fried chicken and mashed potatoes.

If you and your partner are like most of my patients, you may find it hard to resist these and similar tasty treats - foods that, since our childhood, have been associated with feeling good! If you are struggling to get pregnant and perhaps stressed in many areas of your life, comfort foods may hold even greater appeal.

But what might really surprise you to learn is that many of the most well known and delicious "comfort foods" can also boost your fertility!

Indeed, many of the components of some of our favorite dishes can have both a direct and indirect impact on getting pregnant – with many of these foods able to maximize and optimize your ability to conceive.

But before you head for the kitchen for that juicy burger and plate of fries there's something else you should know: Not every "comfort food" is equally nutritious – or good for your fertility.

So, how do you know what to eat and what to avoid when trying to get pregnant? Choosing is easy, once you know just a few simple basics about the three food groups found in many "comfort food "dishes. I'm talking about proteins, healthy fats and carbohydrates - the virtual "trifecta" of not just comfort foods, but pre conception meal planning!

Indeed as important as the phytonutrients found in fruits and vegetables are to your health and your fertility, without at least some of the nutrients found in a selection of healthy fats, complex carbohydrates and proteins,   getting pregnant could still be more difficult than it has to be.

But when you combine the power of these three food groups with the power of fruits and vegetables you not only have a balanced diet that will impact your overall health in many positive ways, you'll also have the basic dietary guidelines that studies have shown can maximize and optimize your fertility as well.

To help you discover all this and more,   the next stop on our Fertility Food Train takes us to the butcher shop and the fish market - where I'll help you discover some of the ways in which lean beef and poultry along with fresh fish, can give your fertility a super power boost with foods that are easy to prepare and delicious to eat!

Super Protein Power: What to Eat To Get Pregnant

For many years I, and many other fertility experts, have known the secret power of protein to impact conception in a positive way. In my best selling fertility books Getting *Pregnant* – and *Green Fertility* - I have consistently recommended that one of the best ways for a woman to boost her fertility is to increase her protein intake by at least 10 to 12%.

Fertility Foods

As important as fruits and vegetables are for improving your fertility, you also need some of the nutrients found in a selection of healthy fats, lean red meat proteins and complex carbohydrates like whole wheat pasta.

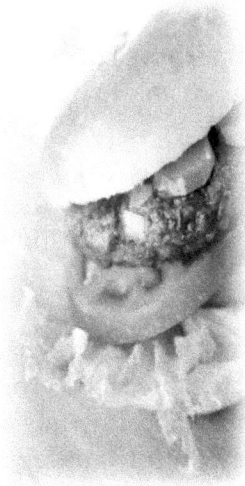

How can this help? A number of studies have shown that when protein intake is insufficient, the hormones which control ovulation may not work as efficiently. Indeed, women who skimp on protein often see disruptions in their menstrual cycle – periods arriving late, early or sometimes a cycle is skipped entirely. If this is happening to you it's a red flag that you may not be eating enough protein.

Conversely, studies show that when protein intake is high, ovulation tends to occur more regularly – which depending on your age, could mean you will have an egg available for fertilization during every cycle. And this dramatically increases your chances for conception.

Moreover, once you do get pregnant, increasing protein intake is even more important, for you *and for your baby*. According to the American College of Obstetricians and Gynecologists, consuming adequate amounts of protein during pregnancy can increase your developing baby's birth weight and that may protect against premature delivery, as well as increase your baby's overall health .

And if you conceive a baby boy – well protein is essential! A relatively new study published in the *Journal of Physiology* found that when protein intake is low during pregnancy, it affects the development of the reproductive system of baby boys.

More specifically, male genitals may not fully develop and/or testicles may not fully descend. Later in life, sperm production may be chronically low, impairing the ability to father a child.

So, making sure you get enough protein during your pre conception period will also help ensure your baby is getting the proper nourishment right from the moment of conception!

But that said, not all forms of protein are equally healthy or equally effective for increasing fertility. And it's important that you learn the difference between different sources, so you can create the meals that will do the most to boost your fertility as well as ensure your baby's health.

Certainly, I have always personally believed that lean red meat is among the best protein sources if you are trying to get pregnant, followed by white meat poultry and fish. And to some extent I still believe this is true.

However, considering some of the newer research on the negative health impact of animal fats found in many red meats, as well as the mercury issues that have arisen regarding fish, several years ago I updated my recommendations to include consuming smaller portions of red meat, poultry and fish, and advising my patients to make up the difference by increasing their intake of plant-based proteins. And I'm happy to report this recommendation was recently endorsed by Harvard researchers studying the effects of various proteins on ovulation.

According to their research women who added just one serving per day of plant –based proteins to their diet - including beans, tofu, soybeans, or nuts - appeared to have fewer ovulation problems then women who ate less of these foods.

Choose Your Proteins Wisely

While I agree with the Harvard findings in terms of the health benefits of eating more plant-based proteins, where my recommendations differ is in the type of plant protein you eat. More specifically, I am not a huge fan of daily servings of soy based proteins if you are trying to get pregnant. The reason?

Soy proteins exert a weak but still significant form of plant estrogen – the same type many women use during menopause to alleviate symptoms of an estrogen deficiency. But in younger women, who do not have an estrogen deficiency – and may actually have an estrogen overload – eating soy foods on a daily basis could throw off the balance of brain hormones linked to egg development and ovulation, making getting pregnant more difficult. And this is exactly what a number of studies have found.

- In one meta-analysis published in the *Journal of Nutrition* in 2002 researchers cited a number of studies in which an increase in soy protein resulted in increased menstrual cycle length and a decrease in estradiol, progesterone and sex- hormone binding globulin – all key biochemicals necessary for conception.

- In a study published a few years earlier in the *American Journal of Clinical Nutrition* researchers found that a high soy intake actually suppressed both LH and FSH – which as you read in Chapter One, are two key hormones necessary for egg production and ovulation.

Now certainly, if you spend even a little time researching fertility on the Internet then you have probably noticed many sites filled with anecdotal stories of women who claim to have regulated their menstrual cycles and improved their fertility profile by consuming large amounts of soy – with some claiming that soy supplements are as good as fertility drugs such as Clomid when it comes to encouraging egg production and ovulation. And if you are over age 35 and your estrogen levels have started declining, or if you have been diagnosed with fertility problems related to a *lack of estrogen*, then yes, these soy foods or even soy supplements can be helpful.

But for women under age 35, the majority of whom are not estrogen deficient, then eating too much soy, or taking soy supplements could be a mistake.

So, how do you know where you stand?

- If you are very thin, if you tend to exercise a lot and if you have highly irregular menstrual cycles and/or you know for sure you are not ovulating on a regular basis, then you could have an estrogen deficiency.

- If, on the other hand you are of normal weight or slightly overweight, and tend to suffer from symptoms of PMS before the onset of each menstrual cycle, then your estrogen levels may be normal or even elevated.

Another way to know for certain is to have your doctor perform either a blood or saliva test to check your estrogen levels. Without clear medical evidence that your estrogen levels are low, I suggest you err on the side of caution and limit your intake of soy foods and particularly soy supplements.

Of course this does not mean you must avoid soy-based foods entirely. Certainly they can be a good way to increase your protein intake without adding more animal fat to your diet. The key is to eat these foods *in moderation* – including soy as just *one source* of plant-based protein, while looking to other sources to fill in the gaps, including beans, legumes and nuts.

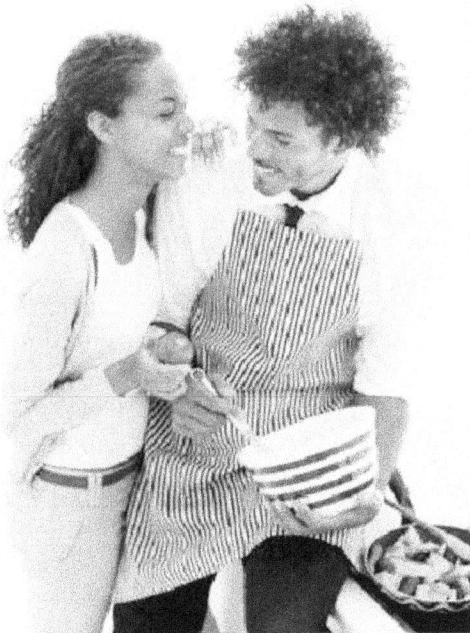

Men and Soy: What You Must Know

As you may have already figured out, any food that acts as a source of estrogen can't be good for male fertility.

And if this is what you are thinking, then you are right to assume soy is not a good choice for men trying to conceive a child.

In the same Harvard research group that found links between soy and female fertility, doctors found also found that men who ate a lot soy based foods saw a reduction in sperm count.

More specifically, after an analysis of all the data in the study – which took into account factors such as a man's age, and his weight - researchers found that those men who consumed as little as a half-serving of a soy food every day (the equivalent of about a half of a soy burger), had on average, 40% fewer sperm than men who did not eat these foods.

Beer, Peanuts & Sperm!

Studies from the Medical Research Council in Cambridge, England found that both beer and peanuts could contain enough plant estrogens to impact sperm count. So while trying to conceive your partner should reduce or eliminate both beer and peanuts from his diet!

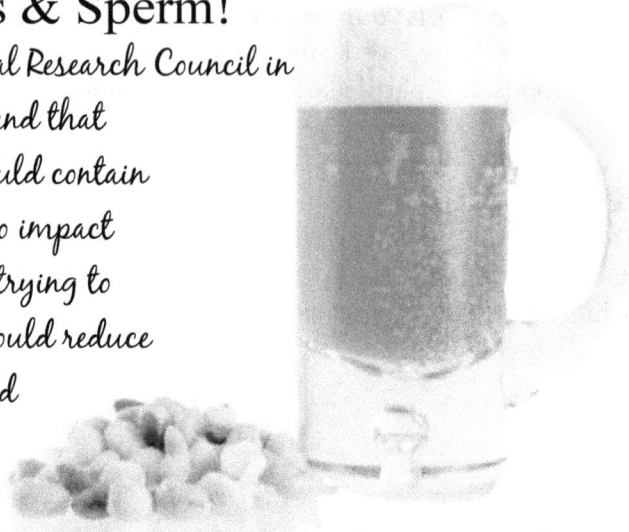

If he just can't give up his nightly brew, then he should limit the amount to no more than 1 mug or bottle of "Light beer" (not dark ale) - and definitely substitute cashews or walnuts for peanuts!

While sperm count of men who ate the soy were still within the normal range, they certainly represented the "low normal" end of the spectrum.

My concern, however, is that if your partner's sperm count is already low due to any number of other reasons, filling his plate with soy-based foods could be enough of a negative assault to drop his sperm count far below normal, making conception much more difficult.

As such, my advice is for men to avoid soy based foods during the time baby making is on the agenda! Also note, however, that it's not just soy that contains plant estrogens capable of impacting sperm.

Other foods he should avoid include peanuts, red wine, and brown ale. As I pointed out earlier, studies from the Medical Research Council in Cambridge, England found all three of these foods contain enough plant estrogens to impact sperm production

Discover A New Fertility Protein

If, in fact, you want to reduce your intake of soy – but still consume more vegetable-based protein- you might want to investigate the benefits of products made from lupin.

Another type of legume with a similar protein profile to soy, it is currently garnering rave reviews in the healthy eating communities.

Grown in Australia and now being milled into flours for bread, rolls and other baked goods, lupin is not only higher in plant protein than soy, it is also high in two types of fiber – both insoluble (like oats) and soluble (like apples).

Since fiber is key to helping control blood sugars – which can also impact fertility in some women - lupin-based products may be a valuable fertility food to add to your daily diet!

Perhaps most important, studies have shown that when compared to soy, lupin is far, far lower in phytoestrogens, to the point where the effect is believed to be minimal to none on hormone levels.

For all these reasons I highly recommend products made from lupin flour as a good source of plant-based protein.

If you can't find products made from lupin flour, check out a brand new product known as Lupin8. A soluble, flavorless powder that can be used in everyday cooking, Lupin8 combines the health and dietary benefits of lupin kernel flour (LKF) resulting in a product that is high in dietary protein, fiber, omega-3s, folate, niacin and is rich in antioxidants – all important for fertility.

Another bonus: Lupin8 also helps you feel full ! For those who are looking to lose some weight in order to increase fertility Lupin8 can help you do that.

For a super powerful fertility protein breakfast add Lupin8 to your morning cereal.

For lunch, add it to soups, stews, casseroles or homemade bread – you won't taste it and it won't change the texture.

Or you can try combining it with whole wheat flour, dark chocolate and walnuts for a home-made fertility-boosting brownie! (Check out our recipe at FertilityDietGuide.com)

Ice Cream:
The Ultimate Comfort Food Could Help You Get Pregnant!

One of the most delicious forms of protein – not to mention the comfort food on the top of everyone's list - is ice cream. And while we don't normally think of this food as necessarily healthy – let alone being a fertility booster – the truth is that for some women it can be both!

How can it help? First, as I just mentioned, ice cream is a powerful source of dairy protein. But as good as that is, in the past we were all discouraged from eating ice cream due to its high animal fat content. Not only can this pack on the pounds, as you will learn in the next section, animal fats can be bad for your health and bad for your fertility.

So why is ice cream the exception to the rule? The very latest research indicates that certain high fat dairy products – particularly ice cream and milk - appear to have some protective effects on ovulation, effects that, for *some* women, override the negative influences of the animal fat. In research conducted by Harvard University, doctors found that one or two weekly servings of whole milk as well as foods made from whole milk— such as ice cream, full-fat yogurt, or cheese – can, in some women, reduce the rate of ovulation – related fertility problems.

Conversely, these same products made from low- fat milk had the opposite effect, increasing ovulation problems.

So what is it about high fat milk products that make them so good for fertility? Many believe the link can be found in estrogen. More specifically, estrogen and other reproductive hormones are stored in fat – not only in humans, but also in animals, particularly cows. So when milk – or milk byproducts such as ice cream or cheese – is fully fatted, they contain an abundance of these hormones.

But remove the fat from the milk – and you no longer have these extra hormones. In older, post menopausal women this reduction is a good thing since too much estrogen in the post menopausal years can increase the risk of certain cancers. But some researchers now believe that for women in their childbearing years with ovulatory problems related to an estrogen deficiency, the "extra" hormone boost you get from high fat products can be helpful.

As such, if you suspect an estrogen deficiency exists, and particularly if your doctor confirms that this is true, then the hormone boost found in full-fat dairy products may be enough to tip the scale from infertile to fertile and help you get preganant.

- According to the Harvard research, the high fat dairy products most likely to encourage conception include whole milk and ice cream.

- The foods most likely to have a negative impact on fertility include sherbet, frozen yogurt and low fat yogurt, all of which appeared to contribute to ovulatory dysfunction – or at the very least did nothing to improve ovarian function in women with low estrogen.

What's more the finding was also dose –responsive: The more low fat dairy products a woman consumed, the more difficulty she had getting pregnant. Conversely, the more full-fat dairy products she consumed – to a point - the less likely she was to have problems conceiving.

Certainly this research is still considered preliminary. Moreover, remember that, like the soy based foods high in plant estrogens, the positive effects on fertility only apply to women not making enough estrogen on their own – including those who may be underweight.

Conversely, if you are overweight, or sometimes even if you are the right weight, you may actually be producing too much estrogen, in which case eating ice cream or other high fat dairy products could contribute to a hormone imbalance that will increase your fertility problems.

Who Needs Ice Cream and Who Doesn't!

Much like my advice concerning soy intake, if you are not overweight and want to add high fat dairy products to your diet in moderation, feel free to do so – but do remember that moderation is the key.

One serving per day of full fat milk, along with two half cup servings of full fat ice cream per week will net the desired effect!

Also be certain to compensate for the extra calories by eating less of other foods - and reducing your intake of saturated fats from other sources, such as red meat.

You should also be vigilant about watching your intake of snack foods, particularly those high in trans fats such as potato chips, French fries and donuts.

Once you do begin adding ice cream to your diet wait two weeks and look for the following signs:

- If your periods become more normal and tests show you are ovulating more consistently – then it's a good indication high fat dairy foods are helping. So you should continue to eat them.

- If your periods become more irregular, or you develop other symptoms of a hormone imbalance – including severe PMS (pre menstrual syndrome), acne, oily skin or hair, or mood swings – then the high fat dairy products may be increasing or even causing a hormonal imbalance and increasing your risk of infertility.

Also remember that once you do become pregnant, you should switch back to low fat dairy products. This will help keep you from gaining excess weight during your pregnancy - which is great for you and healthy for your baby!

Men and Ice Cream

Because of it's link to estrogen, it's a good idea for men to avoid all high fat dairy products while trying to conceive . Because the estrogen content in these foods can definitely impact testosterone dominance, too much full fat ice cream could make it more difficult for his body to manufacture high quality sperm. And this in turn dramatically reduces your chances for getting pregnant.

High fat dairy foods he should avoid include not just ice cream, but also milk and yogurt. Eating low fat dairy products in moderation, however, is fine. Additionally men should have no problems adding sorbets, sherbet or other low at frozen desserts to their diet - as long as they eat it in moderation and are careful not increase the amount of sugar in their diet, which as you will read about later,
can also be bad for male fertility.

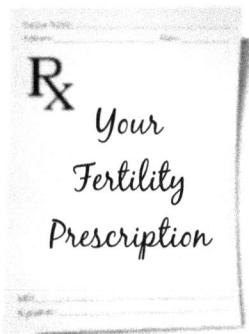

Rx Your Fertility Prescription

Fertility Proteins:
My Personal Prescription

To increase your intake of protein and improve your fertility profile I recommend you and your partner add the following to your weekly diet:

· 3 meals containing fish (salmon, tuna or mackerel are your best choices).

· 2 meals containing eggs, chicken or turkey (white meat only) per week

· 2 meals containing lean red beef per week

· 2 servings of beans per week

· 1 serving of a soy-based food such as tofu or soy milk per week (women only)

· 5 servings of low fat dairy – including yogurt, cheese or milk.

· 2 servings per week of high fat ice cream (if needed).

Comfort Foods & Cravings ....

The Carbohydrate Connection To Fertility

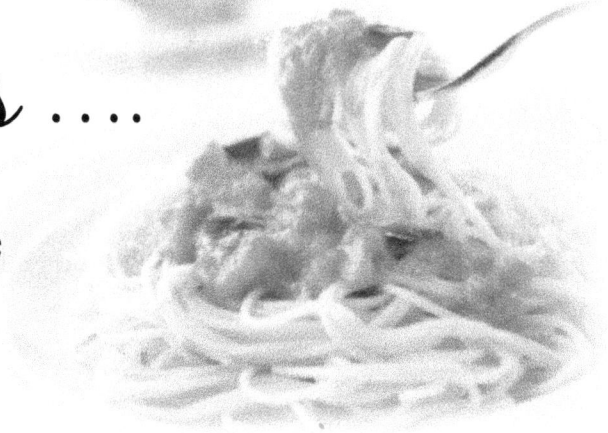

If you're like many women, the days leading up to your monthly menstrual cycle can be filled with food cravings – an overwhelming desire to eat things that normally you might not even favor.

While for some the craving can include a desire for sweet or salty foods, for the vast majority those pre-menstrual snack attacks are representative of just one food group: Carbohydrates. Bread, bagels, cookies, cake, pretzels, pasta, chips – these are just a few of the carbohydrate-rich foods that many women seek out – and some *have to have* - in the days leading up to a monthly period.

If this is starting to sound familiar, then you already have one clue as to how the food group known as carbohydrates can be linked to fertility. In short: The fluctuations in reproductive hormones that occur following ovulation - and grow stronger just before the start of each cycle – are intimately linked to a variety of brain chemicals, at least some of which control both our appetite and our cravings for foods high in sugar and carbs.

Conversely, however, eating these same foods can also have a reverse negative effect, inhibiting the production of brain chemicals necessary for getting pregnant.

The "catch" however is that while some carbohydrates can affect your brain chemistry in a way that encourages fertility, other types of carbohydrates can have the opposite effect , so pregnant is much harder than it has to be.

Learning to tell the difference between which ones have the power to help and which ones can do you harm is your first step in utilizing *this* food group to its best possible fertility advantage.

So how do you know which foods fall into which group? The key to making those choices is a concept nutrition expert's call the "Glycemic Index". In short, this refers to how much sugar is released when certain types of carbohydrates are digested – and for some women it can play an extremely important role in conception.

Good Carbs – Bad Carbs: What You Must Know

As many of you may already know, the word "carbohydrates" is a kind of "umbrella" term under which fall a great many foods. In the first group you find foods such as fruits, vegetables, grains (like whole wheat, brown rice and oats), legumes (like peas, peanuts and soy) and tubers, like yams.

But for most of us, the term "carbohydrate" immediately brings to mind the foods that fall into the second group: Yummy sugar-laden snacks such as cake, cookies, pies, and candy bars as well as "comfort" foods such as bread, pasta, muffins and macaroni made from processed white flour.

The way nutritionists split these two groups is via the terms ComplexCarbohydrates (the first group) and Simple Carbohydrates, (the second group).

Simple carbohydrates are foods that once ingested quickly break down into sugars which are then rapidly released into your blood stream.   These foods are also referred to as having a **"high glycemic index"** – which in simplest terms means they release lots of sugar into your bloodstream soon after eating them. They include items such as cakes, cookies, pies, breads, pasta and muffins.

Essentially items that contain lots of processed white flour (which is metabolized as sugar) as well as lots of sugar itself. So it's easy to see why they release large amounts of sugar into your blood stream soon after eating them.

The other group of carbohydrates is known as "complex carbs". This group includes foods such as fruits, vegetables, and whole grains – and overall, they react quite a bit differently in your body. Indeed, they are called "complex" because digestion takes a lot longer – thus, the release of sugar into your bloodstream is slow.

For this reason these foods are also known to have a **"low glycemic index"** – meaning their release of sugars is less and much slower.

So now you may be asking yourself what does all this have to do with getting pregnant? The answer lies how your body metabolizes or "handles" **a "glycemic sugar load".**

How Sugar Affects Fertility

The link between a **food's "glycemic index"** and fertility begins with a hormone known as "insulin". This is a natural chemical secreted by your pancreas after every meal (Your pancreas is a small organ located in the middle of your abdomen). The purpose of insulin is to remove the sugars from that meal that are now floating in your bloodstream, and carry them into your cells. Here, your body converts the sugars into a source of energy that gives you the "get up and go" you need every day. If you eat more sugar than your cells can hold, the remaining surplus is stored in your liver and is released gradually as your body's demand for energy increases.

But more than just moving sugar from your bloodstream to your cells, insulin has still another job. It acts as kind of "door knocker" that literally instructs each cell to "open up" and let the sugars in. Moreover, because "simple" or "quick burning" carbohydrates – like white bread, or sweet cake or cookies – are quickly converted by your body into sugar soon after eating them, your pancreas is forced to produce a lot of insulin in a very short time – and to quickly begin the "door knocking" process that signals cells to open up and take the sugar.

When you eat quick-burning, sugar-laden foods *only occasionally*, or you eat them in very small portions, this rapid release of insulin isn't much of a problem.

Over time however - or when you eat a lot of these "quick burning "carbs - the picture can change. Indeed, the more of these foods you eat and the more insulin that is constantly being released into your bloodstream, the more often your cells are bombarded with insulin's "knock". And the more often this occurs, the less responsive your cells become – which means that more insulin is required each time to get them to open up and let the sugars in.

When you reduce your intake of simple carbohydrates and replace them with complex carbohydrates like fruits and vegetables, you and your partner gain protection from some of the major diseases of our time, as well as improve your fertility!

When it gets to a point where your body is continually being forced to put out greater and greater amounts of insulin just to clear sugar from your bloodstream, a condition known as "insulin resistance" can develop. If not treated and the diet not changed, this condition is a precursor to type II diabetes – wherein your cells become so resistant to "insulin's" knock that it requires medication to help clear the sugar from your blood.

But long before this happens, the wear and tear of insulin resistance begins to show up in what may seem like an unlikely area: Your reproductive organs. Indeed, the more insulin your body is forced to produce, the greater the potential impact on your fertility. How and why does this occur?

Because insulin is a hormone, its part of a finely tuned network of balanced biochemical activity at least some of which is involved in egg production and release. So, as you might imagine, when your body is forced to continually put out greater and greater amounts of insulin, suddenly that finely tuned network can begin to go somewhat out of balance.

Like an orchestra with a single violin that is out of tune, when your body has even one hormone that is out of sync with the rest of the network, it throws off the entire pattern of production – including the production of reproductive hormones necessary for getting pregnant.

In fact, over time, the entire hormonal network necessary for conception can be affected, leading to a number of fertility problems. Among the most common involves an increase in the production of androgens, male hormones such as testosterone.

Normally, your ovaries produce tiny amounts of testosterone. And in small amounts it can have some very advantageous effects, including increasing your sex drive and even your "baby making lust"!

When however, insulin levels are consistently high – as they are when you eat a lot of "simple carbs" – it sends a message to your ovaries to step up testosterone production – which in turn also slows down or even halts estrogen production.

The end result: The brain chemistry necessary to signal both egg production and release goes entirely off course. Not only does the low estrogen/high testosterone ratio mean your eggs will have a hard time developing, but even if they do, ovulation may not occur.

But to what extent can your fertility be affected by a diet high in these "quick burning" simple carbohydrates? According to one study women who consumed the highest level of quick burning simple carbohydrates were a whopping 92% more likely to experience ovulatory infertility than women who ate less of these foods! And this held true even after the researchers considered other factors that could impact fertility, such as age and smoking.

The Carbohydrates That Hate Sperm!

While the link between fast burning carbs and female infertility has been proven time and again, it's important to point out that this is not strictly a female problem. Indeed, over the last several years studies have begun to uncover links between male fertility and blood sugar levels - so much so that we now know that eating a diet high in simple carbs can have an overwhelming impact on the entire hormonal network necessary for healthy sperm production.

In one meta-analysis on the topic of male infertility recently published in the *Journal of Andrology,* doctors reported that insulin resistance as well as type II diabetes are major contributing factors in a condition known as "hypogonadism" – which in simplest terms means testicles that simply don't produce enough testosterone. Since the testicles are the "factory" where sperm are made, when function goes down, and testosterone production falters, sperm production plummets.

As the study also pointed out, insulin resistance appears to have a direct connection to not just low testosterone, but also impaired spermatogenesis (which is the creation of healthy sperm), as well as having a direct effect on sperm concentration and motility.

Insulin resistance in men has also been linked to an increased number of sperm containing damaged DNA. These are sperm that not only have difficulty fertilizing an egg, if they do, the rate of miscarriage skyrockets – simply because the embryo contains the same damaged DNA found in the sperm.

The Carbohydrates That Can Help You Get Pregnant

After reading all this information on the negative effects of carb-rich foods, you may be thinking that the best way to get pregnant fast is for you and your partner to just stop eating carbohydrates altogether.

But this would be a mistake. Indeed, your body and your brain can't really function without carbohydrates – it's the fuel that helps us think, gives us energy and helps keep that finely balanced network of fertility hormones humming along. Sound like a contradiction to what you just read? It's not. Because it all has to do with the type of carbohydrates you and your partner choose to include in your diet.

While some – **like the quick-burning, high-glycemic carbs** we just discussed – can clearly have some negative effects on your fertility, the **slow burning "complex carbohydrates"** can have the opposite effect - and even boost your fertility considerably. Indeed, the foods that make up this category – fruits, vegetables and whole grains – have been shown in studies to boost fertility and make getting pregnant easier!

In fact, in the massive Nurses' Health Study researchers discovered that women whose diets remained high in "complex carbohydrates" – particularly fruits, vegetables, and whole grains - decreased their risk of ovulatory-related problems and were able to pregnant faster and easier than women who did not include these foods in their diet.

This finding dovetails perfectly with previous research reporting that most slow burning carbohydrates are also high in fiber - an important non-nutritive compound that not only helps keep blood sugar balanced, but also works to pull heart-harming cholesterol from your blood.

Indeed, the American Dietetic Association has confirmed that fiber is an essential element for controlling blood sugar as well as helping to control weight – two factors that also play an important role in getting pregnant.

And this is particularly important news for men, since studies also show that high cholesterol can impact testosterone production as well as the production of other hormones necessary for healthy sperm production.

In fact, in one study highlighted in the *Journal of Andrology,* doctors reported that high cholesterol had a *direct impact* on semen quality and fertility. The research, which looked at 106 male partners from infertile couples, found 65% had high cholesterol, high triglycerides (another type of blood fat) or both.

So, it's clear that both you and your partner need some carbohydrates in your diet. But, by reducing your intake of simple carbohydrates (foods like white rice, potatoes, and anything made from white flour or sugar) and replacing them with complex carbohydrates (foods such as high fiber whole grain bread and cereals, and plenty of fruits and vegetables) you can optimize your fertility , improve your overall health, reduce your risk of diabetes, and most definitely increase your chances of getting pregnant!

So, what *specific carbohydrates* should you eat to boost your fertility – and which ones should you avoid? On the following page you will find a quick summary to help you make your choices.

But for more information I encourage you to visit FertilityDietGuide.com – our website devoted to healthy eating before, during and after pregnancy.

Or pick up a copy of our book The Fertility Diet Guide, which features information on hundreds of delicious foods proven to help boost your fertility - including the Glycemic Index on over two hundred foods proven to help your fertility.

Carbohydrates & Conception:

What To Eat To Get Pregnant!

While almost any food is safe to eat in moderation, there are certain items that have been shown to have a positive impact on fertility - and others that have been proven in studies to have a negative effect.

To help get you thinking in the right direction here is a quick round-up of the carbohydrates I've found to be most helpful to fertility and the ones that have the potential to do some harm.

The Good Carbs to Eat:

Whole grain bread; whole grain pasta; spelt (a grain) ; oatmeal; buckwheat; barley, brown rice; whole grain cereals like Cheerios, Special K, Complete or Total; fruits such as apples, apricots, blueberries; cantaloupe; grapefruit; and strawberries; vegetables such as cabbage, broccoli; cauliflower; yams; pumpkin; soy beans; lupin; salad and tomatoes.

The Bad Carbs To Reduce or Avoid:

Cake; candy; soda; fruit juices; anything sweetened with high fructose corn syrup; cupcakes; French fries; donuts; white bread; white rice; mashed, boiled or baked white potatoes (cold potato salad okay in moderation); fruit juices; sweetened cereals; rolls; pies; potato chips; pretzels.

Fat Can Boost Your Fertility! What You Need To Know

It wasn't such a long time ago that we all experienced the "fat free" revolution. Everywhere we looked – from magazines and newspapers to our local supermarket aisles – the words "fat free" jumped forward.

The idea behind the movement was that by cutting the fat from our diet – and particularly from yummy items like chips and baked goods – we would experience a collective weight loss and come away much healthier.

Unfortunately, that nutrition experiment flopped! Not only were many of the fat substitutes used in commercial products the underlying cause of a great many gastro intestinal woes, while replacing fats most manufacturers upped the sugar content of their products. And of course the one tenet no one seemed to realize was that "fat free" does not equal "calorie free".

The end result: Not only did we, as a nation NOT experience weight loss, many credit this "fat free revolution" with the real start of the obesity epidemic in this country. We ate more, we took in more sugar, and we disrupted our insulin producing network, and in the process upset our entire hormonal network. Indeed, there is actually a significant correlation between the rise in fertility problems and the advent of "fat free" foods!

But as bad a move as this was, it also helped teach us a very valuable nutrition lesson. And that is, that not all fats are created equal! While some – like trans fats and animal fats – are indeed bad for us, other fats – like those that come from vegetables and plants – are not only good for us, they are essential to good health.

And nowhere is this truer than when it comes to enhancing fertility. Indeed, studies have shown that by reducing your intake of the "bad" fats, while increasing your intake of the "good" fats, it's possible to make a significant and measureable increase in your fertility status. For many couples, this one simple dietary change can, over time, turn them from infertile to fertile. And this is not just true for female fertility, but for male fertility as well.

So how do you know which fats to eat and which ones to avoid? It just so happens that the next stop on our Fertility Food Train is the "Good Fat- Bad Fat" Depot – where I'll help you and your partner decipher the latest nutritional guidelines about fat and discover what to eat to boost your fertility!

The Good Fats That Help You Get Pregnant Faster!

As I just mentioned to you, not all fats are created equal. In fact, even among the "good" or "healthy" fats, some are clearly better than others.

But no matter how you slice the nutritional pie, it's clear that at the very top of the list of the fats most likely to benefit your fertility are those known as MUFAs – short for mono-unsaturated fats.

Derived from sources such as olives, nuts and fruits like avocados, and found in products such as canola oil, walnut oil, grape seed oil and mayonnaise, MUFAs not only help increase your overall health, they can also counter some of the nasty effects of the "bad fats" – including helping to reduce your cholesterol. This is particularly important for male fertility since, as you read a little earlier in this chapter, high cholesterol has a direct effect on sperm and can dramatically reduce a man's fertility profile.

MUFA fats can also help stabilize blood sugar levels and in the process help normalize the hormonal activity necessary for optimum fertility.

But as important as MUFAs are, they are not alone on the fertility pantry shelf! Right alongside them- and of equal value - is another group of healthy fats known as PUFAs – short for polyunsaturated fats.

Among this group are what are known as "essential fatty acids" or EFAs - key factors necessary to maintain healthy cells throughout your body . In fact, EFAs play an even more vital role in your overall good health and your fertility by directly impacting the production of hormone-like compounds that help regulate blood pressure, blood clotting, and blood fats, as well as insulin production.

Most important – at least in terms of your fertility – are two particular EFAs known omega 3 and omega 6 - compounds is that while they are essential to your health, your body cannot manufacture them on it's own. As such, you need to get them from foods or supplements.

And this is one reason why your fertility diet can play a critical role in your ability to get pregnant!

Omega 3's: the Super Fat Fertility Boost

While both omega 3 and omega 6 are important fats to include in your diet, when it comes to boosting fertility, it is omega 3 fatty acids that hold the most significance. In particular two specific omega 3 fatty acids - compounds known as eicosapentaenic acid (EPA) and docosahexanoic acid (DHA) – can make the biggest dietary difference in how quickly you get pregnant.

The greatest food source of these compounds is cold water fish - like tuna, mackerel and salmon. But if you have some concerns over mercury toxicity linked to fish, you can also get these same compounds from flax seed and walnuts, as well as some foods fortified with DHA (and more on this in a few moments).

What's important right now is to know that in whatever form you choose, omega 3 fatty acids will have a direct impact on ovulation, as well as reducing inflammation body-wide, including the kind that frequently leads to fertility-disrupting hormone imbalances.

This is particularly true if you have been diagnosed with PCOS – poly cystic ovary syndrome. In one study published in the *Journal of Clinical Endocrinology and Metabolism* in 2004 researchers found that simply adding more omega 3s to the daily diet had enough of an impact on hormonal production to kick start ovulation in women with PCOS who were not ovulating at all!

Other research has shown essential fatty acids can have powerful anti-inflammatory effects on the fertility-robbing menstrual related disorder endometriosis – and in the process help reverse many of its fertility-robbing effects. (And you can read more about both these conditions and their special dietary guidelines that can help in my book "Green Fertility: Nature's Secrets for Making Babies.")

Moreover, omega 3 also helps protect against some of the fertility robbing effects of a high carbohydrate diet and in particular insulin resistance, in both men and

Striking a balance is key!

As important as Omega 3 fatty acids are, the best   results
come when you strike a balance between foods containing
Omega 3 and those containing Omega 6 .
The ratio to   shoot for is   4 to 1.
Which means you should eat 4 meals
containing omega 3 fatty   acids for every one
meal that contains omega 6 fatty acids!

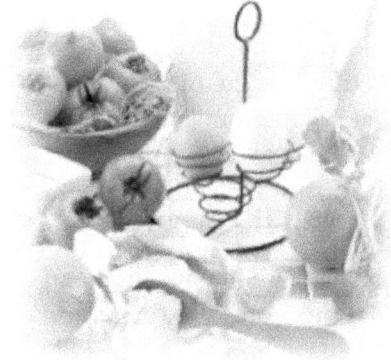

women. So they are not just important for you to include in your diet, but also important for your partner as well.

After you get pregnant, omega 3's help promote your baby's growth and development by increasing blood flow to the placenta – which, in its earliest stages may also help protect against miscarriage.

Moreover, a diet rich in omega 3 fatty acids both before and after you get pregnant can help reduce your risk of premature birth, and may help you avoid preeclampsia (a dangerous rise in blood pressure that can occur during pregnancy) as well as post partum depression.   According to research published in the *Journal of the American Dietetic Association*, eating foods rich in omega 3s during pregnancy can also reduce the risk of gestational diabetes.

And if that were not enough to convince you to add these healthful foods to your diet, studies show that moms who consume lots of heart-healthy omega 3 foods before and during pregnancy may give birth to a smarter baby - with all indications that this compound contributes to brain development in the womb and encourages a higher level of intelligence later in life!

Keep The Balance and Get Pregnant Faster!

As important as omega 3s are to your health and your fertility, you'll derive the most benefits when you combine them, in the proper balance, with omega 6 fatty acids. These are found in foods such as eggs, poultry, most nuts, whole grain breads and cereals, canola oil, soybean oil, corn oil – even the new trendy weight-

weight-loss/health berry known as Acacia are very high in omega 6 fatty acids!

But why is it so important to strike a balance between omega 3 and omega 6?

While omega 6 fatty acids possess powerful anti-inflammatory factors that can aid in getting pregnant, they need omega 3's in order to exert their healthful effects. Indeed, when omega 6 fatty acids outnumber omega 3 fatty acids, they turn from anti-inflammatory compounds to inflammatory ones, upsetting hormonal balances and causing a negative effect on your fertility – as well as increasing your risks of diabetes and heart disease.

Moreover, when your intake of omega 6 rises too high – with no balance from omega 3's - it promotes the formation of blood clots. This not only increases your risk of heart attack and stroke, but also your risk of early miscarriage. In fact I have seen a number of patients who, while believing they could not get pregnant, were actually conceiving, then losing their pregnancy very early on. For many, simply balancing their intake of omega 3 and omega 6 fatty acids helped them overcome early pregnancy loss and go on to deliver healthy babies.

In fact, the very latest research shows that the most promising health effects of essential fatty acids overall are achieved through a proper balance of omega-3s and omega-6s.

The ratio to shoot for: Roughly 4 parts omega-3s to 1 part omega-6s. And this may be easier to accomplish than you realize. Why?

Since so many foods we normally eat are loaded with omega 6, by simply adding 3 fish meals a week to your diet, along with a handful of walnuts and using flax on your cereal or salad several times a week, you'll be getting a great supply of omega 3 – and likely a good balance to the amount of omega 6 you consume.

If you don't want to eat fish note that the omega 3 found in foods like nuts, seeds and grains are not a direct source. Instead they contain a nutrient known as ALA – short for alpha linolenic acid, which the body converts to DHA, the form of omega 3 most helpful to fertility.

While the conversion process happens naturally, a variety of individual health factors, including your nutritional status, can sometimes hamper the conversion process. The end result is your body may get less of the omega 3s than it would if you were in optimum health.

One way around this is to eat more of these foods than you think you need. The other way is to supplement your diet with foods that already contain DHA – so the conversion is done for you!

Currently you can purchase eggs, egg whites, soy milk, whole wheat bread, and cereal fortified with DHA.   To make sure you're getting a product fortified with not just omega 3's but specifically DHA, read the label.

Finally, if you still think you might not be getting enough omega 3s, you can also take a supplement, alone, or in conjunction with the omega-3 rich foods. In a later chapter you'll discover how to select the best omega 3 *supplements* .

The Fats That Can Harm Your Fertility: What You Should Avoid

As good as the "good fats" can be in helping you get pregnant, that's how bad the "bad fats" can be when you're trying to conceive.

So, what exactly are "bad fats" – and which ones should you try to avoid? On the top of the list is saturated fats. These are mostly animal-based fats that come primarily from sources like red meat, processed foods, poultry skin and egg yolks.

How can avoiding saturated fat help you get pregnant faster?

First, saturated fats can increase your risk of insulin resistance, which as you read earlier, contributes to infertility in various ways.

But more than that, saturated fats also increase the production of triglycerides. These are a byproduct of saturated fat that is stored in your cells after you eat a meal high in fat – like that big juicy steak or steamy hamburger and fries.

Besides increasing your risk of heart attack and stroke, studies show that triglycerides can have a direct impact on fertility.

Indeed, in one recent study published in the journal *Human Reproduction*, doctors suggested that a diet high in saturated fats can directly impact the production of key reproductive hormones, and slow down the overall functioning of the ovaries, thus contributing to problems getting pregnant.

When you replace the "bad" fats in your diet with "healthy" fats
You not only help your heart but you also help your fertility!

There is also some evidence to show that these "bad fats" can reduce the number of egg follicles (the seeds from which your eggs are made) while also impacting the hormones necessary for ovulation. This also increases your risk of infertility.

Moreover, some very new and interesting research also published in the journal *Human Reproduction* suggests that the saturated fat you do eat can go directly to your eggs which in turn prevents them from being fertilized - even with the help of sophisticated fertility treatments such as IVF.

Indeed, after analyzing eggs that failed to fertilize, the researchers found the majority contained higher-than-normal levels of saturated fat!

The good news however, is that by reducing your intake of "bad fats" and whenever possible replacing them with the "good fats" we talked about earlier, you can have

Trans Fats and Your Fertility

In addition to the problems associated with saturated fats, a second "fertility enemy" can be found in a type of manufactured compound known as "trans fats".

These troubling compounds occur during the conversion of liquid oil into a solid shortening – the type used in many commercial baked goods and fast foods in order to extend their shelf life. The problem is that while these hybrid shortenings may extend the life of the foods on supermarket shelves, the trans fats that result do the opposite for those of us who consume them. In short, tran's fats are now believed to be a direct link to heart disease, insulin resistance, type 2 diabetes – and now, infertility.

Indeed, in one study recently published in a leading nutrition journal researchers found that women whose diet included just 4 grams of trans fat per day had a whopping 93% more fertility-related ovulation problems.

How does the damage occur? Many believe trans fats incite inflammatory reactions within the body that impact hormone production and may also affect the interior of your fallopian tubes. When inflammation lines the tubes they can not only make it harder for sperm to survive, they also make it harder for an egg to be fertilized or for the resulting embryo to survive.

Because trans fat also impacts the way sugar is metabolized in the body, they can sometimes act similar to quick-burning carbohydrates, increasing your risk of insulin sensitivity. As you read earlier this can impact ovarian function, but in particular, egg production and release.

Moreover, my personal research and experience has also shown that trans fat may be a contributing factor to the menstrual related disorder known as endometriosis, the leading cause of infertility among young women. If this is a problem you're already dealing with, then cutting trans fats from your diet will not only help reduce your symptoms, but may even help you gain better control over the condition in general.

So, how do you cut trans fats from your diet? The easiest way is to read food labels on every packaged food you buy. Indeed, thanks to new FDA guidelines, all commercially available foods must disclose their level of trans fat.

Read The Label!

If you take just a little time out when shopping to read the labels you'll know instantly how much trans fat a product has . You should try to consume no more than 4 grams of trans fat total for the day.

The goal for you and your partner is consume less than 4 grams of trans fat a day each - and the lower that number can go, the better it will be for your fertility.

But while reading food labels and "counting" up your trans fat grams; I want to pass on a few words of warning: Labels that say "No Trans Fat "are not always what they seem!

Legally a food can contain up to one-half gram of trans fat per serving and still carry the label "trans fat free". Since we all know that serving sizes are deceiving (studies show most of us automatically double the serving size, particularly when eating prepared foods) , it's easy to see how you can easily consume 4 grams or more of trans fat a day, even if you think you aren't getting any!

Add to this the foods that you know contain significant trans fats and you eat them anyway – such as French fries or a doughnut – and it's even easier to hit or even surpass that fertility-robbing 4 grams of trans fat a day and still believe you are eating healthy.

So, again, it's important that you aim for the lowest possible number of trans fat grams daily. I promise you that doing so will definitely be worth the effort and that effort will be reflected in not only better health overall, but also a better fertility profile overall, for you and your partner.

Feed Your Fertility…

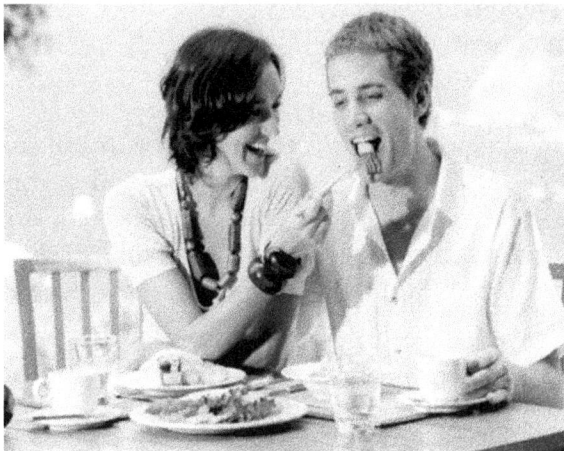

& Nurture The One You Love !

While I'm hopeful the information in this chapter can help you to understand more about the importance of a healthy diet, the real take home message, from me to you and your partner, is for both of you to eat as healthfully as you can, but not to worry.

While your diet can certainly play an important role in helping you get pregnant, if you are filled with worry and fear over what you are eating, the resulting stress will work against the good dietary choices you do make. As you will learn later in this book, stress can be a major contributing factor to infertility, so you don't want to overload your circuits with worries about eating the right foods. Just do what you can to improve your diet and heed as many of the precautions as your lifestyle allows.

But even more importantly, I hope you will use your meal times, especially dinner time and weekend meals, to share some relaxing moments with your partner. Too often I see couples living in a rushed, "gotta do it now" world, where dinnertime is literally "on the back burner". Take out foods, processed frozen dishes, snack foods that we eat on the run, in our car, standing at the kitchen counter or while hovered over a computer - none of this is good for your digestion or your fertility! Instead, I propose that you take a moment to   not just stop and smell the roses, but stop and smell the scent of fresh foods on your dining room table – and to share the love of those foods with love for each other, turning every meal into a meaningful, shared experience.

If you can also prepare the meals together, you'll each know and understand which fertility foods are good for each other – and encourage each other to eat more of them, even if your meals involve some pre-cooked or fast foods once in a while. If you can also use your dinner hour as a time to share some positive and meaningful conversation together, I can promise that the benefits of your healthy menu will be magnified!

Indeed, far too often I see couples who don't recognize the importance of sharing a relaxed, happy, meal together – and to do so on a regular basis. This is particularly true for those couples for whom the idea of "trying to conceive" becomes one more thing on their already overloaded "To Do "list.

But if you can use your dinner hour, and hopefully some meal times over the weekends as a shared positive experience – a time when you and your partner can relax together and really enjoy not just your meals but the time you are spending together, you will not just garner the benefits of healthy eating, but you will also receive emotional benefits that can have a powerful impact on all your conception efforts.

I guess what I am really saying is that if, while you are taking the time out to nurture and feed your body with healthy foods, remember to also take some time to "feed and nurture" the love you and your partner have for each other. Because in the end, that's really what feeding your fertility is all about!

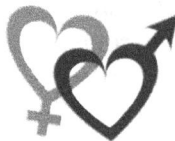

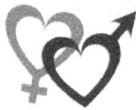

Chapter Four

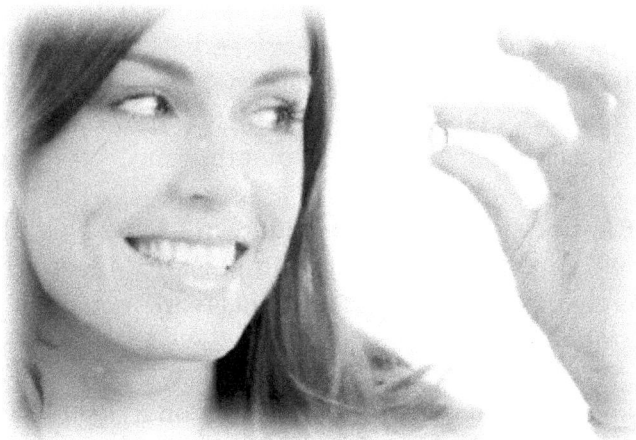

The Fertility Power Boosters:

It's Vitamin Supplements!

While we often don't think of vitamins as "medicine" – and certainly not as "fertility drugs" - more and more we have come to see that in many ways vitamins and other nutrients can and do play an amazing role in healing the body and enhancing health, including the ability to get pregnant.

In fact, one of the factors that makes *healthy foods* so *healthy* are the dozens of healing and helpful nutrients they each hold inside. While science has identified some of these compounds, many are yet to be discovered. In fact, one of the most powerful aspects of a healthy diet is that all the factors - known and unknown - work together in a synergistic fashion to bring about some amazing results, particularly when it comes to getting pregnant.

This is why I have always believed that the power of nutrition lies more in whole foods than it does in isolating individual nutrients.

But that said, there are certain key vitamins and minerals that, on their own, have also been linked to fertility – and in some cases can act almost like a "fertility drug" to enhance the chance of conception. While these same nutrients are also found in foods – and of course, in my mind, this remains their most powerful source - still, it's often impossible to eat all of the foods necessary to get the kind of nutritional boost that vitamins and minerals can supply.

For this reason I do recommend that you enhance your healthy diet with a number of key supplements - vitamins that science has shown, (and I have personally witnessed) have important effects on fertility. In some cases, where a severe enough vitamin deficiency exists, simply adding these supplements to your daily diet is enough to turn you from infertile to fertile in just a few months time.

But even if you're just a little under the nutrition radar and have only slight deficiencies, I have found that, in combination with the powerful foods I have recommended in the previous chapters, these same nutrients work incredibly well to impact your fertility in a positive way.

So without further ado I'd like to take our Fertility Food Train on a *slight* detour - one that will help you discover the vitamin and mineral supplements that will personally work best with your fertility diet. Doing so will help enhance the health of you and your partner and in the process also maximize your pregnancy potential!

Understanding Vitamins

Just one flip through any magazine or online health site and its' easy to see that vitamins are making headlines worldwide. Never before have we had the kind of research available to show the power that certain nutrients have to make a significant difference in our lives.

But while it may seem as if vitamins are a "new " health craze, the truth is, as far back as the 1800's scientists began to understand that certain nutrients found in foods could make a difference in our health. In fact, the very first vitamin "on record" is thiamine or vitamin B1. The groundwork was laid for this discovery by a Scandinavian physician named Dr. Christian Eijkman who, at the time was caring for patients in the Dutch West Indies, all victims of an epidemic "disease" they called

"Beriberi". The symptoms included fatigue, irritability, abdominal pain and eventually changes in nerve transmissions that eventually resulted in a deadly degeneration of muscles, including heart muscles.

In an effort to find a cure for Beriberi, the hospital research lab maintained a flock of chickens used for various treatment experiments. Normally the chickens were fed what they referred to as a "cheap brown rice", while the more "prized" white rice was fed to the patients and the staff. At one point, however, the hospital ran out of brown rice and started feeding the chickens the white rice. And what happened? All of the chickens began exhibiting symptoms of beriberi disease.

Now if you're thinking "poison rice" - well not so fast! Because ultimately what Dr. Eijkman gleaned from this situation was that the white rice created a kind of nutritional deficiency that resulted in the symptoms linked to beriberi. And moreover, that brown rice seemed to protect against that deficiency. Indeed, once the chickens were put back on a diet of brown rice, all their symptoms disappeared! It was at this point that Dr. Eijkman was the first to conclude that the "disease" called "beriberi" wasn't a disease at all – but simply the result of what they then called a "food deficiency."

It wasn't however, until 1911, that a polish researcher named Casimir Funk was able to identify the substance in brown rice that could prevent the symptoms of "Beriberi". He determined that the "chemical" belonged to a category of organic molecules known as "amines". He believed that amines were "vital" to human health – and thus he named the isolated compound a "Vitamine". Later the name of that compound was changed to "thiamine" – which we now know as B1, the first vitamin to be discovered. Eventually the nutrient category was changed to the word "Vitamin" – without the "e".

In the years that followed, additional nutrient compounds continued to be identified and all of them linked to symptoms of deficiencies that were once thought to be diseases – including "scurvy" , a condition also attacks muscles and bones can be cause by a Vitamin C deficiency.

 Today we are not only still isolating and identifying new nutrients in foods, we're also discovering new ways that these nutrients can improve our health . And nowhere is this truer than when it comes to fertility!

Indeed, researchers are continually uncovering new and important links between conception and nutritional status – *in both men and women.* Certainly, in my own medical practice, where I have helped thousands of couples conceive and deliver healthy babies, I have seen first-hand the power of many of these nutrients to not only increase fertility but to help bring into the world healthier, stronger, even smarter babies. In fact, based on my own personal research as well my personal experience with patients, I continued to recommend nutritional supplements even when there was only a glimmer of evidence proving the impact.

Today, I am proud to say that much of what I have always believed to be true about the power of vitamins has been *proven* true in study after study – with some of the research conducted at the biggest medical centers and universities in all parts of the world. And in this chapter I'll bring the most important of these studies to your attention.

At the same time, however, I still want you to keep in mind that supplements are exactly that – *supplements*, which means "in addition to" your daily diet. So never use them in place of healthy eating, or believe that simply taking a vitamin pill cancels out your need to eat healthy or live a healthy lifestyle!

In fact, I can't tell you how many patients have come through my office doors believing that all they had to do to compensate for a lifetime of bad habits was pop a vitamin pill! As I always told them – and I tell you now - while it's true that certain vitamin supplements do have amazing restorative powers, it's also true that the most positive and beneficial effects can be seen when your diet and lifestyle are healthy as well.

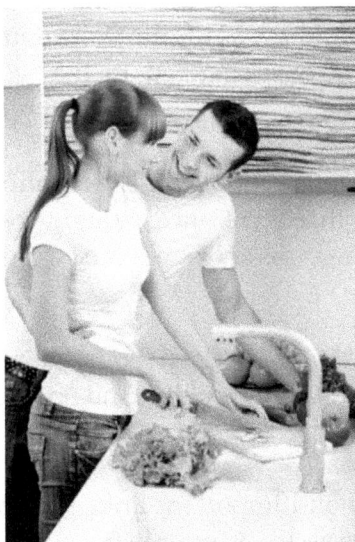

Super Fertility Nutrients: The Vitamins You Both Must Have!

One of the most important factors that allow vitamins to boost fertility is a concept known as "synergy". This is a powerful natural network that allows all key nutrients to work together in a way that increases their individual power even more.

In fact, the power of synergy is so strong that isolating a single vitamin or a single mineral and taking only that one supplement is the quickest way to create deficiencies of other important nutrients.

One way to insure this doesn't happen is for you and your partner to lay your nutritional foundation with a high quality multi-vitamin. For you this can come in the form of a pre-natal vitamin, and for him it should be a multi-vitamin developed for men.

Taking these supplements every day is key to making sure that you each get a well rounded and complete source of nutrient support for your entire body. Indeed, one of the best and most important ways to boost your fertility is to begin by boosting your overall health - and certainly a multi-vitamin is a good place to begin obtaining that boost!

But that said there are also a number of key nutrients that have been shown to impact both male and female fertility - so it's also important to include these in your regimen as well.

While some have been shown in studies to have specific effects on certain aspects of fertility – such as ovulation in women or sperm production in men - others have been shown to work in consort to tone and improve the reproductive system as a whole.

Depending on the multi-vitamin you choose, some of these nutrients may be included in your daily vitamin supplement already   – though usually in lesser amounts than what is necessary for specific fertility needs.

When this is the case it's usually okay to add an additional supplement to what is already in your multi vitamin to increase its potency even more. When it's not okay to go beyond a certain level, I'll let you know that, so that your supplement intake is always health giving and in the proper balance.

Super Fertility Nutrient # 1: Folic Acid

When it comes to both boosting your fertility as well as insuring your baby's health from the moment of conception, no nutrient is more important for a woman than folic acid.   Also known as Vitamin B9, folic acid is essential to the production of red blood cells for both you and your partner. However, when it comes to conception this vitamin holds special significance for you – particularly if you suspect you may not be ovulating on a regular basis and want to protect against more serious ovulatory –related problems.

Indeed, in one study involving more than 18,000 women those who took a vitamin supplement high in folic acid dramatically reduced their risk of developing ovulation-related fertility problems. Moreover, the effect was dose-related. In short, the more folic acid a woman consumed, the lower her risk of fertility problems.

Folic acid is also important if you have a history of miscarriage and/or you are at risk for very early miscarriage. Indeed, many patients have come to me believing they could not conceive, when in reality I discovered they were actually getting pregnant, but losing their babies at such an early stage, they didn't even know they had conceived. When this is the case I find folic acid to be an extremely important and helpful nutrient, with the amazing ability to help embryos survive and thrive.

And, in fact, this was also the finding of one major collaborative research project between the NCHID in the United States and the Karolinska Institute in Sweden. Publishing their findings in the *Journal of the American Medical Association*, the researchers suggested that the earlier you begin taking folic acid, the greater your chance of avoiding miscarriage.

But taking folic acid during your pre conception time also benefits your baby. How? We have long known that when used during pregnancy, folic acid supplements reduce a baby's risk of neural tube defects, a serious congenital malformation that is also a leading cause of infant death.

Indeed, the National Institute of Child Health and Human Development (NICHD) reports that the simple act of adding 400 mcg of folic acid to your diet during your pregnancy dramatically decreases your baby's risk of developing both brain and spinal cord defects. In fact, even adding as little as 100 mcg of folic acid a day is enough to reduce your baby's risk of birth defects by some 22%.

But how can folic acid help *before you conceive?* First, it is imperative that your baby receive all the benefits of folic acid right from the very moment of conception. You could, in fact, easily be pregnant 4, 6 or even 8 weeks before you know it – and waiting until your pregnancy is confirmed to start this nutrient could actually deprive your baby of important benefits in the first critical 6 to 8 weeks of life.

Moreover, because so many factors in our daily lives deplete folic acid, it can be easy to fall short of this nutrient. Certain oral contraceptives, cholesterol medications, and drugs used to treat Poly Cystic Ovarian Syndrome and type II diabetes, common pain relievers like aspirin and ibuprofen, and most antibiotics can all deplete folic acid. So, even if your diet is healthy you could still end up with a deficiency. For this reason it's imperative that you take adequate folic acid supplementation, starting as soon as you decide you want to get pregnant.

Share A Fertility Salad!

Make a salad brimming with vegetables rich in folic acid like spinach, asparagus & Romaine lettuce with just a dash of wheat germ!
Then, enjoy it together!

Other Foods High In Folic Acid Include:

Fortified breakfast cereals (up to 400 mcg per serving); half cup of boiled spinach (100 mcg); 4 spears of asparagus (85 mcg); ½ cup chopped broccoli (50 mcg); I ounce of dry roasted peanuts (40 mcg); ½ cup Romaine Lettuce (40 mcg); 2 tablespoons wheat germ (40 mcg); 6 ounces tomato juice (35 mcg); ¾ cup orange juice (30 mcg); ¼ cantaloupe (25 mcg); 1 medium banana (20 mcg).

While multi-vitamins and particularly pre-natal vitamins are a good start, I also recommend that you increase your dosage over and above what these provide. (See below).

Folic Acid and Male Fertility: A true "couples" vitamin, not only is folic acid important for you, it's also a key nutrient for your partner. Why? First it is necessary for the production of healthy sperm. But equally important it's also key to the overall health of your partner's entire reproductive system. In fact, this nutrient is so essential that a deficiency of folic acid can cause an immediate impact on sperm motility as well as lead to greater production of abnormal sperm. To increase absorption and get maximum benefits it's best to take folic acid with vitamin C.

My Personal Folic Acid Recommendation: To enhance your fertility and give your baby the best possible start in life, I recommend a supplement containing 800 to 1,000 mcg of folic acid daily beginning as early as 6 months prior to when you want to get pregnant – for both men and women.

Super Fertility Nutrient # 2: Beta Carotene/ Vitamin A

When it comes to getting pregnant, there is perhaps no single nutrient more important than vitamin A. Why? Not only is it necessary for the creation of a healthy embryo, when a deficiency does exist it may be impossible to create an embryo strong enough to survive the implantation process. So in this respect, it's easy to see why this nutrient is known as the "fertility vitamin".

One way to ensure you are getting enough vitamin A is, of course to take a vitamin A supplement. But an even better way is to take a supplement known as "beta carotene" - the compound that your body *uses* to manufacture its own supply of vitamin A. Why is this a better approach?

First, beta carotene is one of a number of compounds known as "carotinoids", which as you read earlier, have numerous important health benefits. But when it comes to fertility, carotinoid supplements play a much more important, and specific role.

To begin with, carotinoids are essential to developing healthy follicular fluid, the liquid that surrounds and nourishes your egg. When carotinoids are in short supply and follicular fluid is inadequate, your egg will have a difficult time developing – which means it may not be strong enough or healthy enough to survive fertilization.

Furthermore, even if your egg does manage to develop to the point where it can be ovulated, without adequate beta carotene your brain won't receive the signal necessary to release LH (luteinizing hormone), the compound necessary to trigger ovulation. And without this, your egg wont' be released and ovulation will not occur. Indeed, I have personally seen a number of patients with highly irregular ovulation get their cycles back on track and achieve much more regular egg production and release simply by adding more beta carotene to their diet – either in the form of foods or supplements, or a combination of the two.

But as important as this is, there is still one more reason to take beta carotene supplements: And it has to do with insuring a healthy uterine lining, one that can support and nourish your fertilized egg. Indeed, once your egg is ovulated the "shell" it leaves behind is called the "corpus luteum" - and it immediately begins manufacturing progesterone.

As you read earlier, this is the hormone that, together with estrogen, helps turn the lining of your uterus into a soft, spongy "nest" or "womb" where your newly

How Beta Carotene Affects Your Fertility

The corpus luteum is the empty shell your egg leaves behind after ovulation. It's job is to manufacture progesterone & get your uterus ready for implantation.

Because the corpus luteum is made up largely of beta carotene, when levels of this nutrient are low, progesterone production may falter. When it does your uterine lining may never fully develop, so your fertilized egg may never get a change to implant deep enough to continue growing. ut by insuring beta carotene levels remain high, you can help ensure that you are giving your newly

fertilized egg can implant, develop and grow. The more spongy your uterine lining is, the better the chance that your fertilized egg *will* attach and begin growing – and the more likely it is that your pregnancy will be successful.

Conversely, the thinner your uterine lining is, the weaker it is – and the less likely it is that your pregnancy will continue. In fact many women who are plagued with recurrent miscarriage are actually deficient in progesterone – meaning their uterine lining never becomes quite thick enough or strong enough to "hold" onto a fertilized egg.

So, how does this all tie in with beta carotene? The corpus luteum shell is largely made up of beta carotene! As such, when levels of this nutrient are low, progesterone production may falter – and when it does your fertilized egg may never get a change to fully implant and grow. But by insuring beta carotene levels remain high, you can help ensure that you are giving your newly fertilized egg the very best possible chance for survival.

While some of these same effects can be garnered from taking vitamin A supplements as opposed to beta carotene, I don't recommend that you make this switch. Why?

Once you are pregnant, excess levels of vitamin A have been found to increase the risk of certain birth defects. In fact, the American College of Obstetricians and Gynecologists recommend that vitamin A supplements should never exceed 770 mcg daily (or 2, 567 International Units).

Because, however, you may be pregnant up to 8 weeks before you know it, it's a good idea to watch vitamin A intake before pregnancy as well as during pregnancy. With beta carotene however, you won't have this problem, since it is entirely safe to use both during and after pregnancy. So that's another reason to make beta carotene your vitamin A supplement of choice during your preconception time.

Indeed, when you analyze all the benefits, it seems that getting your vitamin A from a carotene supplement - instead of a vitamin A supplement - offers the best possible advantage for you and your baby.

When shopping for a beta carotene supplements, however, do be certain to choose a product that contains *the full complement* of carotinoid nutrients and not just beta carotene alone. Not only will all the compounds work together to bolster your fertility, there is some evidence to show that doing so may be healthier for your body overall.

If, however, you choose to take a vitamin A supplement, make certain that it does not exceed the ACOG recommendation of 770 mcg per day – or 2,567 international units.

IMPORTANT TO NOTE: While vitamin A from supplements can build in the body and eventually cause a toxic overdose, beta carotene appears to not have this effect, so generally supplements are safe. However, at very high doses (30 mg or more) there are some risks, so make sure to speak to your doctor before taking any super potent supplements.

Beta Carotene and Male Fertility: Simply put, it is impossible for a man's body to produce testosterone if he is short on vitamin A! Since testosterone is key to sperm production, if the supply of this hormone is even a little bit under par, sperm count can plummet. Moreover, the number of abnormal sperm also increases thus increasing the risk of miscarriage. Additionally, key compounds found in beta carotene make up 1/3 of each sperm – so when this nutrient is in short supply, sperm definitely suffer. As an antioxidant, beta carotene also works to protect sperm against free radical damage – which in turn means more healthy sperm available for conception. And finally, beta carotene it is also an essential nutrient for the health of the seminiferous tubules, the area of a man's reproductive system which helps sperm to mature.

My Personal Fertility Recommendation: Supplements containing up to 25,000 international units of beta carotene daily, in a supplement that also contains other carotenoids including lycopene, lutein, and alpha lipoic acid for both men and women.

Foods High In Beta Carotene Include: Carrots, sweet potatoes, yams, apricots, winter squash, pumpkin, cantaloupe, and mangoes. Other good sources include dark green leafy vegetables such as kale, collard greens, spinach, leaf lettuce and broccoli. Interestingly, your body can utilize the beta carotene in these foods best when they are cooked, chopped or pureed.

Foods High In Vitamin A Include: Whole or fortified milk, fish liver oils, tuna, shrimp, salmon, liver, eggs, some varieties of cheese.

Super Fertility Nutrient # 3: Vitamin B6

As part of the group of nutrients known as B complex, doctors have long known that vitamin B 6 (pyridoxine) plays an important role in many aspects of women's health.

First isolated in the 1930's, we were quick to discover that this water–soluble vitamin interacts with over 100 different enzymes, and in doing so is linked to many key chemical reactions in the body. This includes improving the functioning of red blood cells, as well as influencing activity of your nervous system and your immune system.

It wasn't however, until many years later that we also began to forge links between B6 and fertility. And the first clue came when researchers made connections between this nutrient and PMS – pre menstrual syndrome.

More specifically, research revealed vitamin B6 has a direct connection to the production of both serotonin and dopamine, two brain chemicals best known for their link to mood and behavior - including some symptoms of PMS. But what you may not realize is that both serotonin and dopamine are also part of the finely tuned biochemical network of brain hormones necessary for conception. As such, when levels of either serotonin or dopamine go out of balance, you can not only experience greater anxiety and depression during your premenstrual time, but also experience an imbalance of other hormones necessary for conception.

In fact, because serotonin has a direct impact on both FSH (follicle stimulating hormone) and LH (luteinizing hormone) in both men and women, many believe it can also have a direct influence on the daily activities of both male and female reproductive organs.

More specifically for you, serotonin can influence everything from egg production, to maturation, and release, as well as play a role in the subsequent production of progesterone necessary to turn your uterus into a spongy "nest" that will nourish your embryo.

What's important to realize, however, is that the ebb and flow of not just serotonin and dopamine, but many brain hormones is influenced by levels of vitamin B6. Indeed, when a B6 deficiency occurs, not only is serotonin production compromised, but so is the related brain chemistry necessary for egg development and ovulation.

How do you know if you are deficient in B6? For many women the most outstanding symptom is a whopping case of PMS! Despite some recent studies showing that B6 may not be as important to PMS as once thought, I can tell you from my personal, clinical experience that B6, particularly in balance with vitamin B complex, can and does help many women control their symptoms of PMS and in doing so also help control the subsequent hormonal imbalances that are the underlying factor in many cases of infertility.

But it's not just the connection to PMS that makes B6 an important fertility nutrient. Indeed, this nutrient has also been found to help your body control blood sugar levels. What's the connection to fertility?

As you read earlier, when sugar can't get into your cells (a condition known as 'insulin resistance') it initiates an entire cascade of hormonal activity that ultimately impacts ovulation in subtle but important ways. Indeed, I have personally found that many instances of "unexplained infertility" can frequently be traced to this subtle impact of blood sugar levels on ovulation.

In fact, as I previously reported in my best selling book "Getting Pregnant: What You Need To Know Now", studies conducted as early as 1979 revealed that women who were diagnosed with "unexplained infertility" appeared to benefit from taking between 100 mg and 800 mg of vitamin B6 daily.

B6 & Male Fertility

As important as B6 is to your fertility, it is just as essential to your partner's fertility. In fact it's not only necessary for the production of testosterone –the sperm making hormone – when a severe B6 deficiency exists your partner may not be able to produce enough healthy sperm for conception to occur.

In fact, one of the first signs of a B6 deficiency in men is a low sperm count – and if your partner has been diagnosed with a low, or even low-normal sperm count then it's a sure bet he's also low in vitamin B6 – and he must take steps to replenish his body immediately. In animal studies, a prolonged deficiency of B6 has resulted in complete infertility.

Fortunately, however, even a severe deficiency is easy to correct – and sperm react quite quickly. Within a few weeks of taking high potency B6 supplements. sperm count can rise substantially, along with an increase in the number healthy sperm available for conception.

While the study was small and in no way considered conclusive, I can personally tell you that I have also helped many women diagnosed with "unexplained infertility" to conceive within several months via a combination of dietary changes and increasing their intake of B6 in balance with B complex.

One more key fact you should know: As essential as Vitamin B6 is to your health and your fertility, your body cannot manufacture this nutrient on its own. It must be obtained from dietary sources, or from supplements.

My Personal Fertility Recommendation: For women and men, 200 mg - up to 500 mg daily. However this vitamin should always be taken in conjunction with a minimum of 100 mg of B complex, which is a combination of all the key B vitamins. For best absorption, men should always take B6 with the mineral zinc (more on this important male fertility nutrient later in this chapter).

Foods High in B6 include: Fortified breakfast cereals - ¾ c (up to 2 mg per serving); Baked Potato - flesh and skin, 1 medium (up to .70 mg) Banana, 1 medium (.68 mg) Garbanzo beans, canned, ½ c (.57 mg) Chicken breast, cooked, ½ breast (.52 mg) Oatmeal, instant, fortified, 1 packet (.42 mg).

Super Fertility Nutrient # 4: Vitamin B 12

For many people Vitamin B 12 is known as the "energy nutrient" – the vitamin that gives you a blast of instant "get up and go" and helps you avoid fatigue. While this does hold some truth – B12 *is* the nutrient that supplies life-giving oxygen or energy to our cells – when it comes to getting pregnant it has a whole new and different purpose.

First, a B12 deficiency has a direct impact on ovulation, causing egg production and release to slow down and become erratic – which in turn makes it much more difficult to get pregnant.

But because B12 is also crucial to normal cell division – which is how a fertilized egg develops into an embryo – when your supply of this nutrient is low, your fertilized egg may not develop properly, or may not even develop at all.   And because B12 is also crucial to a healthy uterine lining,   if a deficiency exists your embryo may not implant normally or even be able to grow.

If this sounds like it might also increase your risk of miscarriage, you are right – and the link to that occurrence is "homocysteine", another compound produced naturally in the body. Under normal circumstances, homocysteine is converted by the body into various amino acids necessary for a variety of natural, healthy functions.   But what make this conversion possible are the B vitamins, particularly vitamin B12.   So, when B12 is in short supply, homocysteine levels begin to rise.

So what's the link to miscarriage?   High homocysteine levels promote the development of blood clots. When, early in your pregnancy these clots occur in the small capillaries in your uterus, it can prevent the development of your placenta, the sac that surrounds your baby and through which they will receive all their nutrients. Without an adequate placenta, an embryo cannot survive and sadly, the end result is often a miscarriage.

But by keeping B12 levels on par, you also help keep your homocysteine levels under control, which in turn also reduces your risk of miscarriage.

What makes all of this particularly important is that a B12 deficiency is much more common than people realize – particularly if you are a vegetarian, or if you eat very little red meat, which is a major dietary source of B12. Deficiencies also frequently occur if you have even mild digestive disorders, or more serious digestive-related medical conditions such as Crohns or Celiac disease. In all instances B 12 levels can drop significantly with little or no warning signs.

Complicating matters further: Some common factors can mask a deficiency. This includes a diet high in folic acid, which is recommended for getting pregnant!

Taking Vitamins: Make It A Team Effort!

Because we hear so much about the importance of women taking pre-natal vitamins - even before conception - we sometimes forget that men, and male fertility, need vitamin supplements too!

So I encourage you and your partner to not only take your vitamin supplements every day but to make it a team effort! Remind each other - and look after one another - and you'll be boosting your fertility in more ways than one!

Many women deficient in Vitamin B12 are also misdiagnosed as having an iron deficiency and subsequently treated with an iron supplement. This further masks some of the symptoms of B12 deficiency such as fatigue.

But the really comforting news is that preventing a B12 deficiency is easy. Eating foods such as lean red meat, or the white meat of chicken or turkey can definitely help. But equally as important is taking a B12 supplement - and doing so can quickly turn your pregnancy odds around!

In one study published in the *Journal of Reproductive Medicine* women with a history of up to 7 consecutive miscarriages were treated with vitamin B12 for several weeks. Once normal levels of this nutrient were achieved, all the women were able to successfully *conceive and deliver* healthy babies. For several, the B12 resulted in an immediate pregnancy, with a full term delivery of a healthy baby within 9 months!

Indeed, correcting even a mild B12 deficiency can not only give your fertility an immediate boost, but also help insure your pregnancy is healthy and that your baby has the best possible chance to grow and thrive.

For this reason I strongly recommend that you consider taking B12 supplements beginning at least a few weeks before attempting conception. If you are already having problems getting pregnant, ask your doctor about a test to measure B12 levels – and certainly do so before starting any fertility treatments. Sadly, a vitamin B 12 deficiency is often overlooked even by infertility specialists, causing many couples to experience months or even years of failed fertility treatments when in reality all they really needed was vitamin B 12.

Vitamin B 12 and Male Fertility: When the level of this vitamin is low men can experience not only an overall reduction in sperm count, but the sperm that are produced are frequently "poor swimmers" – meaning they may not find their way to an egg quickly or easily enough for conception to occur. A deficiency of B12 can also result in an increased number of abnormal sperm, which can also make conception difficult. In fact, I believe this nutrient is so critical for men they should supplement this vitamin even if their sperm count is considered low-normal or normal. Since sperm production is easily affected by lifestyle factors such as fatigue, a poor diet, stress or even a simple cold or flu, B12 will help insure that even if production slides, it will still remain well within the normal range.

My Personal Fertility B12 Recommendation: For women, 500 mcg daily; for men, 3 to 4 mg daily.

Foods High In B12 include: Three ounce servings of : Clams (84 mcg) mussels (20 mcg) ; salmon (2.4 mcg) beef (2.1`mcg); chicken and turkey (0.3 mcg); egg (0.6 mcg); milk – 8 ounces (0.9 mcg); brie cheese (1 ounce – 0.5 mcg).

Super Fertility Nutrient # 5: Vitamin C

Although you might think of Vitamin C as the nutrient that primarily helps you avoid those winter colds and flu, what you might not realize is that it's also a powerful fertility nutrient for both men and women.

Indeed, vitamin C has a special "affinity" for the reproductive organs – the ovaries in women and the testes in men. In fact, this vitamin actually accumulates and collects in these organs, which is the first clue that maintaining adequate levels is important to the overall functioning of the reproductive system.

In a few minutes you'll learn about how and why Vitamin C can impact sperm production. But right now I want to concentrate on how vitamin C affects *your* ovaries – and how a deficiency can lead to infertility. And it all begins with the process of ovulation.

Indeed, every time you make an egg and it pops through the lining of your ovary, a tiny opening results. In order for the reproductive cycle to continue that opening has to be healed and sealed. Although this is an automatic process generated by the ovary itself, the healing doesn't occur entirely on its own. It requires a number of key compounds, one of which is vitamin C. In fact, without adequate amounts of this nutrient, the healing process could not occur. If it doesn't, the natural cycle of ovarian function can comes to a halt. So, it's easy to see why keeping levels of Vitamin C high can be so important to getting pregnant.

But as important as this process is to conception, there are still more ways that Vitamin C can help you – and it's all about the antioxidant properties of this nutrient. Indeed, as you learned earlier, antioxidants are necessary for fighting free radical damage - assaults on your cells that can interfere with egg development and release. In fact, without some form of free radical protection, eggs would be damaged almost as soon as they come out. Many could not even survive the ovulation process.

But by keeping vitamin C levels optimized you can insure that your body always has the antioxidant protection necessary to naturally keep egg production healthy, and help guarantee they remain healthy as they grow and develop.

But there's still more reasons to supplement your pre conception diet with vitamin C. Studies show that that this nutrient is also present in follicular fluid – the semi-solid liquid that surrounds your eggs and helps them grow and develop. When vitamin C is in short supply, so is follicular fluid – and that can dramatically alter the cycle of growth and development of a healthy egg.

Conversely, when vitamin C levels are adequate, follicular fluid is plentiful – and that means your eggs have a much better chance of not only developing, but also being fertilized. In fact, studies show that taking vitamin C supplements can actually enhance the egg-making benefits of clomiphene citrate, or Clomid, a drug commonly used to help women produce more eggs in conjunction with fertility treatments such as in vitro fertilization.

Perhaps more importantly, when it comes to getting pregnant, the level of vitamin C itself found within follicular fluid also appears to make a dramatic difference in how quickly you conceive. In one study of women undergoing IVF treatment for infertility, doctors found those who took 500 mg of vitamin C daily had the highest levels of this nutrient in their follicular fluid.

Moreover, the researchers also found that the eggs of the women who had successful pregnancies were much higher in antioxidant capacity that those eggs which failed to be fertilized. Again, this tells us that when you take vitamin C you give your eggs some special "fertility armor" to fend off free radical damage. This result is not only healthier eggs, but a healthier conception overall!

Finally, in a study published in the journal *Fertility and Sterility* in 2003, a group of Japanese doctors offered important evidence that vitamin C has the ability to correct what is known as a "luteal phase defect" - a common endocrine disorder that causes a deficiency in progesterone during the second half of the menstrual cycle. As you recall, progesterone is manufactured by the shell your ovulated egg leaves behind, and it's necessary for the creation of a spongy, yet strong uterine lining.

But what happens when, due to a luteal phase defect progesterone levels are low? Not only does your uterus fail to develop a strong enough lining to allow your embryo to implant and grow, but this can be a direct cause of early pregnancy loss. In fact studies show that in up to 5% of all women dealing with chronic miscarriage, the cause is a luteal phase defect.

The good news is that taking vitamin C supplements can completely turn this problem around! In the Japanese study doctors found that just 750 mg of vitamin C daily increased progesterone levels by up to 53%. More importantly it also significantly increased the rate of pregnancy while reducing the rate of miscarriage. And this might be of special interest to those of you who find it's taking longer than "normal" to get pregnant. Why?

As I mentioned earlier, many women who believe they cannot get pregnant are actually conceiving, but miscarrying very early on – sometimes before the pregnancy can even be measured on a test. When this is the case, vitamin C may be especially helpful in preventing that early miscarriage.

So, while we are far from having conclusive evidence that vitamin C can, on its own, increase fertility, there is certainly enough research to suggest that taking supplements can improve not only your chance of getting pregnant, but also ensure that your resulting embryo is strong and well developed enough to thrive.

Certainly, in my own practice I have seen this nutrient make a significant difference in the ease with which many of my patients get pregnant. For some, it was the key factor that tipped the scales from fertile to infertile. For others it helped increase the success of their fertility treatments. And for some lucky women – those in their 40's and long past their reproductive prime - simply taking vitamin C in consort with the other nutrients and following a healthy diet, was enough to bring about a natural conception, even after other doctors told them their only hope was donor eggs.

My point is, if this nutrient can help so many women overcome dramatic fertility circumstances, just imagine the powerful fertility boost it can offer you!

Double Your Fertility!

When you combine the power of Vitamin C supplements with the power of foods high in this nutrient - like delicious oranges & luscious strawberries - you double the effects!

So remember, don't just take your vitamins! Take your vitamins *and* continue to eat foods high in all the important fertility nutrients.

When you do, you'll double your chances of getting pregnant faster!

Male Fertility And Vitamin C

As one of the most critical nutrients for male fertility, a deficiency of vitamin C causes a direct decrease in sperm count and impacts sperm motility . This means your partner not only has fewer sperm, but those he does have may have difficulty navigating through your reproductive system and reaching your egg on time. Moreover, when a vitamin C deficiency is severe enough, sperm actually "clump" together, making it impossible to fertilize an egg.

Vitamin C is also a powerful antioxidant necessary to protect sperm against many forms of environmental damage – problems that can lead to not just abnormal sperm, but abnormal DNA in sperm – which is then passed on to the baby. In fact, studies show that when a man is deficient in vitamin C, any conception that does occur is at higher risk for some serious birth defects. So, the higher the level of exposures he has to environmental factors such as pesticides, chemicals, pollution and tobacco smoke, the greater his need for more vitamins C.

Fortunately, treatment with vitamin C works quickly. In one study published in the *Annals of the New York Academy of Science,* doctors found that after one week of daily doses of 1,000 milligrams of vitamin C, sperm counts rose by some 140%.

My Personal Fertility Recommendation: For women, 500 mg twice daily. For men, 500 mg up to three times daily.

Foods High In   Vitamin C include: Orange juice (6 ounces, 75 mg), Grapefruit juice (6 ounces – 60 mg); Orange, (1 medium 70 mg) Grapefruit (½ medium 44 mg), Strawberries (1 cup, whole 82 mg); Tomato (1 medium 23 mg) , Sweet red pepper (½ cup, raw chopped 141 mg); Broccoli (½ cup, cooked 58 mg) , Potato (1 medium, baked 26 mg).

Vitamin D: A Fertility Boost From The Sun!

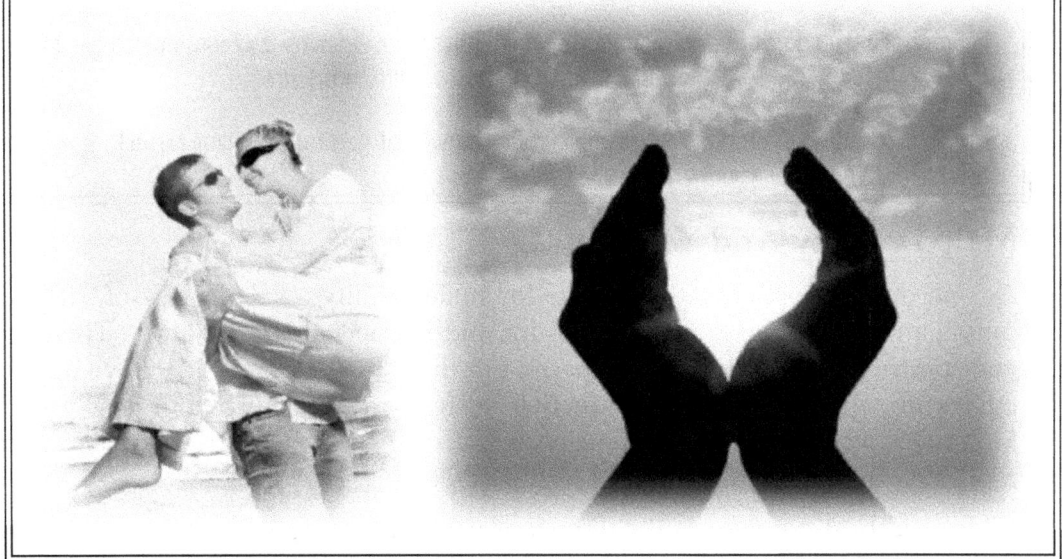

Super Fertility Nutrient # 6: Vitamin D -

Although Vitamin D is known as a "vitamin", in truth, it's really a hormone that your body makes when you are exposed to sunlight. This is one reason why it's known as the "Sunshine Vitamin ."

Indeed, when you feel the soothing warmth of the sun hit your skin, there's a actually a localized chemical reaction taking place – one that produces a natural chemical compound which goes straight to your liver, which then converts it into vitamin D.

This is why it is so important to get at least 20 minutes of sun exposure daily –without sunscreen. And it's not only perfectly safe to do so, it's vital to not just your fertility but your overall health.

But when you can't get that sun exposure – and in many areas of the world it's not possible year-round – then vitamin D supplements can offer a real boost to both your overall health and your fertility.

How Vitamin D Affects Fertility

What makes Vitamin D such a critical fertility nutrient is that it has a direct impact on the reproductive organs –particularly your ovaries. Here, it works to regulate how estrogen is utilized in order to make sure that your egg follicles mature and grow strong.

Studies show Vitamin D also plays a role in how estrogen acts in the uterus, particularly in regard to development of the lining. When vitamin D is not in good supply, it's more difficult to develop that soft spongy lining necessary for your embryo to attach and grow.

So between helping your body make stronger, better eggs, and helping the lining to grow, Vitamin D appears to help reduce the risk of early miscarriage.

But that's not the only way in which this important nutrient impacts your fertility.

One of the ways in which your body maintains proper levels of FSH and LH – the hormones that promote both egg production and release - is through blood levels of calcium. Since vitamin D is critical to regulating and controlling blood calcium levels, it's also critical to maintaining proper hormone levels necessary for conception.

Indeed, without adequate amounts of vitamin D, calcium levels can easily go out of sync – which in turn can impact the production of both FSH and LH, and of course, keep you from getting pregnant.

In fact, one group of Yale researchers studied 67 women who had problems conceiving – and found that 93% of them were low in vitamin D.

According to researcher Dr Lubna Pal, " Of note, not a single patient with either ovulatory disturbance or polycystic ovary syndrome demonstrated normal Vitamin D levels; thirty-nine per cent of those with ovulatory disturbance and thirty-eight per cent with PCOS had serum [vitamin D } consistent with deficiency. "

In another study, women who lost their monthly period altogether and were infertile due to Poly Cystic Ovarian Syndrome were able to kick-start a normal menstrual cycle and get pregnant simply by increasing their intake of vitamin D.

But there is still another link between calcium, vitamin D and fertility –and it has to do with PMS.   Indeed, in studies conducted by University of Massachusetts researcher Elizabeth R. Bertone-Johnson, ScD, and published in the *Archives of Internal Medicine*, we learned that the rate of PMS is significantly lower in women who have a high dietary intake of both calcium and vitamin D.

In fact the study showed that women who ate just four servings a day of calcium-rich low fat dairy or yogurt, or drank orange juice fortified with calcium and vitamin D,

Calcium, Vitamin D and PMS!

Suffering with PMS? It might be due to a hormone imbalance that's also keeping you from getting pregnant.

But good nutrition can help both PMS symptoms and improve fertility!

What to eat: Studies show just four ½ cup servings of vitamin D fortified low fat dairy (like yogurt or skim milk) daily, or two 8 oz glasses of orange juice fortified with calcium and Vitamin D daily could reduce your symptoms of PMS and help you get pregnant!

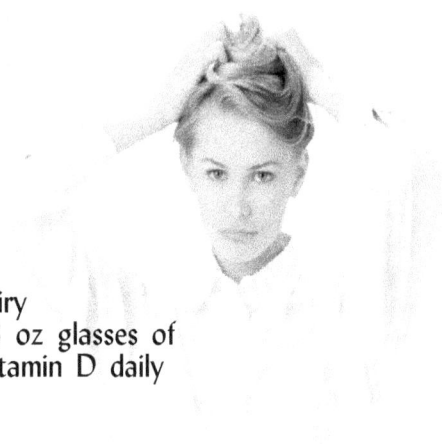

were 40% less like to experience PMS!

So what's the connection to getting pregnant? First, when PMS is under control you will simply feel better with far less stress – which in turn means that all hormone activity will be better balanced. But more importantly, since PMS is a condition underscored by a reproductive hormone imbalance, reducing your risk *of this* problem automatically helps insure better hormone activity overall, and this can have a major impact on conception.

Finally, the very latest research shows that Vitamin D deficiencies may be linked to a higher rate of bacterial vaginosis (BV) an intimate infection that occurs when natural bacteria found in your V zone begins growing out of control. It's a problem that impacts up to 30% of all women in their childbearing years –and if left untreated can lead to serious fertility consequences, including a condition known as PID – pelvic inflammatory disease. When this occurs, all the organs in your reproductive system can become damaged, making it very difficult to get pregnant. So, this is one infection you don't want to get out of control.

But even if your BV infection remains local, the germs themselves can harm and disarm sperm keeping it from fertilizing your egg. If you do happen to get pregnant while you have a BV infection, your rate of miscarriage is higher, as well as your risk of premature labor and a low birth weight baby. But keep your vitamin D levels high, and watch your risk of BV go down!

More importantly, by keeping your vitamin D levels high you can help protect against associated fertility problems and in doing so greatly enhance your chances for conception. What's more keeping those levels high is easier than you think!

In fact, even if you already have a deficiency, the body responds almost immediately to any type of vitamin D stimulation – including spending just 20 minutes in the sun for as little as 5 days. If you add to this foods high in vitamin D (see below) and vitamin D supplements (which I highly recommend) you can not only quickly and easily overcome a deficiency, but give a whopping boost to your fertility as well.

Vitamin D and Male Fertility:

For many years doctors believed vitamin D was only important for female fertility. Today however, we know that vitamin D is also a key nutrient for men. In fact it's essential for the production of healthy sperm in a high enough quantity to bring about a successful conception. In one study of nearly 800 men with fertility problems presented before the Fertility Society of Australia, Dr. Anne Clarke found more than one-third of the participants were severely deficient in vitamin D. Moreover, the vast majority of these men also exhibited signs of DNA damage in their sperm. So, if conception did occur, the risk of miscarriage would be higher than average.

Moreover, Dr. Clarke also noted that a significant number of these men also experienced lower than normal levels of folic acid as well as elevated levels of homocysteine. As you read earlier, elevated homocysteine levels cause small blood clots to form in tiny vessels in the body. In women, this can increase the risk of miscarriage. But in men these blockages can not only rob sperm of nutrients necessary to develop and grow, but also contribute to impotence.

My Personal Vitamin D Fertility Recommendations
Women: 4,000 units daily summer and winter.
Men: 4,000 units daily in summer; 5,000 units in winter

Foods High in Vitamin D: There are two dietary forms of vitamin D: Cholecalciferol and Ergocalciferol. These are naturally found in a number of foods and are usually added to milk and sometimes orange juice. It's important to note, however, that other dairy products such as yogurt and cheese are usually NOT fortified with vitamin D. Other foods sources high in vitamin D include: Cold Liver Oil (highest amount); fatty fish such as salmon, mackerel, tuna, sardines and herring; D-fortified milk and cereals; eggs.

Take a Beach Vacation...

...and get pregnant faster ?

For decades – or longer – gynecologists and even some fertility experts have been advising couples to "take a vacation and you'll get pregnant! " This is, in fact, often a first line recommendation if a couple is suffering with "unexplained " infertility – where there appears to be no physical reason standing in the way of pregnancy.

The goal behind the suggestion has always been primarily relaxation. Indeed, as you will discover later in this book, stress and the hormones secreted when you are stressed, can have a direct and immediate impact on fertility in both men and women. And I'm happy to say that for many couples, taking a vacation – and having some relaxing time together – turns out to be the quickest route to getting pregnant.

Now, however, research has shown us there could be yet another, perhaps more "scientific "reason behind why so many couples do get pregnant when they go away, particularly on a vacation to a warm or sunny climate.

And that is the fertility-enhancing effects of the sun! As you just read, vitamin D is made by the body via exposure to sunlight. So, spending time in the sun - and increasing your vitamin D levels - can have an important and sometimes immediate effect on your ovaries, as well as on the production of hormones necessary to get pregnant. So in this respect, spending time in the sun could give your fertility a boost.

But perhaps even more interesting is the potential effect the sun may have on your partner.

In one very early study on sunlight and male fertility, a group of researchers measured levels of testosterone (the male hormone key to sperm production) in a group of men before exposure to sunlight. They then exposed the men's chests to daily UVB light for five days – each day just long enough to cause a slight reddening of the skin. At the end of five days they re-measured testosterone levels.

What did they find? Exposure to the UVB light (the same kind you get from the sun) caused a whopping 120% increase in testosterone production!

More importantly, they re-measured the levels again 8 days later – during which time the men received no UVB exposure – and their testosterone had dropped down to pre-testing level.

Of course to be totally fair, I have to add that no one has ever attempted to duplicate the results of this study, so we cannot say for certain that sun exposure will increase a man's fertility, or do so this quickly or dramatically.

However, I can tell you that much the way vitamin D helps orchestrate egg development in your ovaries, it plays an equally important role in your partner's testes, where sperm is made.

Adding a bit of epidemiologic fuel to this sun power is data showing that in countries where the latitude is the highest and sun exposure varies dramatically during the year, researchers documented conception rates are highest in late summer (following a season in the sun) and birth rates are highest the following spring!

So, will a vacation in the sun help you get pregnant? There is no guarantee. But, if you combine the romance of the moonlight with the power of vitamin D from the sun....it could happen!

Vitamin E and Your Fertility: What You Should Know

Throughout the years we have seen the popularity of Vitamin E wax and wane. At its height it was considered the "ultimate" vitamin that protected us from heart disease, cancer, and even infertility.

As time went on and more studies were conducted, Vitamin E lost a bit of it's luster. Some of the earlier health claims were disputed and some new concerns arose. And there for a while the "popular" nutritionists seemed to shun the idea of recommending anything more than a minimum daily requirement.

So where are we now? Clearly, the vitamin E pendulum has swung both ways, but the end result has brought us to a nice comfortable middle ground in terms of the power of this nutrient. What has been proven: Vitamin E, particularly when taken in conjunction with Vitamin C remains a powerful antioxidant – and therein lays one powerful link to both male and female fertility.

As with other antioxidant vitamins it is a strong warrior in the battle against free radical damage, plus it also has anti-inflammatory effects. So, for those of you battling borderline insulin resistance, or even if you're just slightly overweight, vitamin E can help control some of the inflammatory factors that might otherwise interfere with your fertility.

But there's another, perhaps even more important link between vitamin E and getting pregnant – and it centers on your cholesterol levels. Indeed, some interesting animal research has shown that when a female's cholesterol levels are abnormal, egg production and quality are affected. In one study published in the *Journal of Clinical Investigation* researchers noted that by simply treating the females with cholesterol-lowering medication, they were able to restore normal egg production and fertility – and they could get pregnant.

But as you read in Chapter Three this could be even more important for men, since studies show high cholesterol can also have a metabolic rebound effect that impacts both testosterone levels and sperm production.

Since vitamin E is key to keeping cholesterol under control, it can have an enormous impact on how quickly and easily you get pregnant.

But more importantly, when levels of Vitamin E drop to the point of deficiency, not only do the testicles begin to degenerate, but the ability to manufacture sperm can come to a complete halt.

The good news: When vitamin E is plentiful, studies show that not only is sperm heartier, healthier and more plentiful, but that egg penetration is more successful. And this means vitamin E supplements may be especially helpful for those couples who suffer with "unexplained" infertility, since one cause is often difficulty in sperm getting into an egg.

My Vitamin E Recommendation
100 units daily for both men and women. If you have cholesterol problems (or a strong family history of this problem) you can safely take up to 600 units a day – as long as you are not taking any blood thinners. If you are, or if you suffer with a very heavy menstrual flow, talk to your doctor before going above the Recommended Daily Amount of 30 units a day. Your partner can safely take up to 800 units a day, particularly if he has been diagnosed with low sperm count, or any sperm abnormality

Four Super Nutrients For Male Fertility!

In addition to the vitamins already mentioned, there are a few additional nutrients that studies have shown – and I have personally seen – make a big difference in male fertility. Remember, up to 50% of all causes of infertility are sperm-related, so it's important that you and your partner work together to ensure your nutritional status as a couple! Indeed, by working together towards your pregnancy goals you not only help ensure that each of you do what is necessary to maximize your fertility, but you'll also develop an important sense of shared responsibility that can boost your fertility is subtle but important ways! To this end, here a few more nutrients your partner should consider taking.

1. Amino Acids - Necessary for sperm production, these building blocks of life can literally help sperm to develop and mature. One particular amino acid known as L-arginine has been known to be particularly helpful for male fertility.

My Recommended Dosage: 500 mg per day of l-arginine. However, your partner should not use these supplements if he has a history of the herpes virus, as this may increase the risk of a break out.

2. Selenium - This mineral is so key to male fertility that if deficiencies go on long enough complete infertility may result. Indeed selenium helps ensure the production of normal-shaped sperm in sufficient enough quantities for conception. It also plays a key role in maintaining the health of the epididymus, the area of the male reproductive system where sperm matures and is held before final release. In one study published in the *Archives of Andrology* we also learned that vitamin E and selenium improved the ability of sperm to swim - a skill necessary to reach the egg.

My Recommended Dosage: 75 mcg per day

3. Zinc - Believed to be the predominant "male nutrient", zinc is critical for everything from the metabolism of testosterone, to the growth of the testicles themselves, to sperm production, motility and count. Zinc also helps suppress excess estrogen in the male body, particularly from environmental exposures.

That said, every time a man ejaculates he loses about 5 mg of zinc. So if you and your partner have a very active sex life, then it's highly likely he is zinc deficient. Moreover, since alcohol, coffee and high fiber foods also deplete zinc it's easy to see how quickly a deficiency can occur.

But it's a deficiency easy to fix! In one study published in the journal *Fertility and Sterility* men with fertility problems who took a daily dose of just 66 mg of zinc in combination with 5 mg of folic acid for only 6 months, increased their sperm count by a whopping 74 percent!

My Recommended Dosage: Up to 100 mg daily

4. Coenzyme Q10 - Present in large amounts in seminal fluid, research indicates that this nutrient works to energize sperm, increasing the ability to swim through a woman's reproductive system and reach her egg.

There is also research showing fertilization rates rise when Coenzyme Q10 supplements are given to men whose partners are undergoing the fertility procedure known as ICSI.

My Recommended Dosage: 200 mg per day

5. Glutathione - A molecule made in the body from three major amino acids - L-glutamic acid, L-cysteine and glycine - together they offer a powerful antioxidant punch. Glutathione is necessary for the formation of a protein that enables sperm to swim.

My Recommended Dosage: 500 mg per day on an empty stomach

Some Final Words:
Vitamins and Diet Are An Inseparable Couple

As I mentioned to you at the start of this chapter, it is my long held belief that eating healthfully is the real key to maintaining a strong and healthy body and a healthy fertility profile.

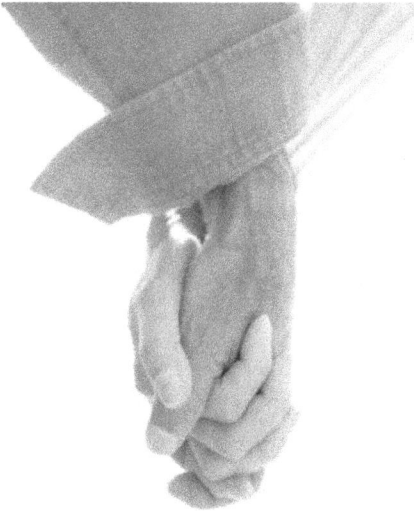

And even though I am offering you information on the power of individual vitamin supplements to boost your fertility, I hope you will remember that a vitamin pill is never a substitute for a good diet. Why?

While we have some very good research on the power of supplements in boosting fertility, they pale in comparison to the impact you can get from whole foods.

For example while the vitamin C extracted from an orange can offer you many healthful benefits, there are dozens, if not hundreds of other compounds found inside the whole orange itself that will benefit your health in many more ways. While some of these compounds are identified, many still remain a "mystery".

What we do know, however, is that by combining the power of whole foods with the power of vitamin supplements, you get the best of what each has to offer. Like an inseparable couple they complement one another and in the process you and your partner reap the nutritional and reproductive rewards!

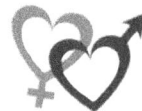

Chapter Five

Nature's Recipes For Boosting Fertility:

The Herbs & Supplements That Can Help You Get Pregnant

I've always believed that one of the truly amazing things about nature is that for every problem, there seems to be a natural solution. Sometimes the solutions are simple – like the blessing of rain to nourish and revive a dying plant or flower. And when necessary, of course, those solutions can be much more complex. But the key thing to remember is that nature always takes care of its own!

this isn't the case. Everything from the stresses of modern living to the effects of the environment, to our nutritional status and more, can come together to impact our reproductive system and make "what comes naturally" much more difficult to achieve.

But the good news is that Mother Nature did not desert you! In much the same way she cares for her beloved plants, flowers and trees, so too are there natural solutions for many of the problems couples experience on the road to becoming parents. For this reason, the next stop on our fertility journey is a health food store – a place where you can not only find wonderful things to eat, but also wonderful natural supplements that science has shown can help you and your partner overcome many of the disadvantages of modern living – the ones that impact fertility.

While these natural preparations can't solve every fertility problem – and certainly not every formulation is right for every couple - amongst the most popular ones, I believe there is something that can help boost the fertility and maximize the pregnancy potential for every couple trying to conceive.

And so, as we go forward with this chapter, I invite you to sit back, relax, and open your mind to the wonderful world of natural supplements – herbs, plants and other natural formulations that science has shown can help you get pregnant.

The Natural Fertility Boosters:
Herbs For Female Fertility

While some of Mother Nature's best kept fertility secrets are good for both men and women, there are a few that are specific to women and some that are specific to men. In terms of your partner, we'll get to those in just a few minutes. But right now I want to concentrate on you – and the herbal products that I have personally found, and studies have shown, can make a measurable difference when it comes to getting pregnant.

But before I give you some specifics, I want to remind you again, that no one factor alone is going to go the whole way in helping you get pregnant - including herbal supplements. I wish it was a matter of popping a magic pill and boom – a pregnancy occurs! But in truth, sometimes getting pregnant requires a little bit of tweaking – and sometimes some major changes – in more than one area of life, be it diet, lifestyle, nutrition or even the use of herbal supplements. Also important to remember: The best and most consistent results come when you use natural therapies in harmony with other natural factors that can impact fertility. For example, while a single herb may have some strong fertility potential, that strength can be magnified many times over when you are also eating a healthy diet, getting the proper nutrition in terms of vitamin supplements, reducing the stress in your life, and getting enough sleep – the importance of which we'll discuss later in this book.

You should also purchase the best quality supplement you can afford. This is important since sometimes discount or no-name brands can be contaminated with pesticides that can actually do your fertility more harm than good.

Finally, the point I want to impress upon you most: To use everything you learn in this book in harmony – and for you and your partner to work *together*, to ensure that the changes you make, both big and small, are made together, as a team. It is when your bodies work in harmony with each other, that your fertility can really soar!

And now, without further ado, here is some information on the herbal supplements that I believe can make a difference in your fertility – and how they can help you.

Fertility Booster # 1: Vitex or Chasteberry

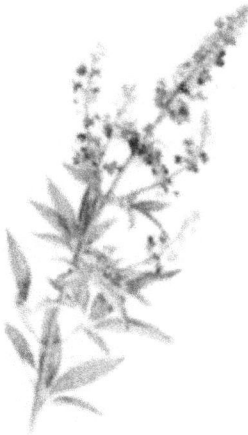

With the botanical name Vitex-agnus-castus-L or "vitex" , this beautiful flowering plant has been used by a variety of cultures around the world as not only a general reproductive tonic, but also a fertility booster. It's power comes from a combination of natural factors including high levels of compounds known as flavonoids – which as you read earlier are prominent in fruits and vegetables. The specific flavonoids found in chasteberry include casticin, kaempferol, orientin, quercetagetin and isovitexin.

In addition, however, chasteberry also contains compounds known as *Spooning glycosides* – natural chemicals necessary in the production of several key hormones. This includes prolactin (related to the production of breast milk) and progesterone, the hormone that is necessary to prepare your uterus for pregnancy and to help your fertilized embryo travel down your fallopian tube to your womb where your baby can begin to grow.

Because of these hormonal effects, Chasteberry is most useful in rebalancing hormones and correcting a condition known as a luteal phase defect – which is a shortage of progesterone following ovulation. In America, many doctors treat this condition with medication. But in Germany, where I first learned about chasteberry, as well as throughout most of Europe, doctors routinely prescribe this herb as the first line of defense for luteal phase defect. Indeed, today the German E commission – which is a lot like the American FDA - believes so strongly in the power of chasteberry to impact hormonal balance, they have approved its use as a treatment for cycle irregularities as well as PMS.

Chasteberry has also proved useful in the treatment of amenorrhea (lack of a menstrual cycle) – which frequently occurs because of a hormone imbalance.

In addition, Chasteberry has also been proven helpful in cases of "unexplained infertility", another problem frequently linked to a hormone imbalance.

But right about now you may be asking yourself, is it all folklore – or does it really work? I'm happy to tell you that numerous new and exciting studies have shown that chasteberry has indeed been proven to work.

- In one recent 3 month study of just under 100 women with either a lack of a menstrual cycle or a luteal phase defect, doctors found that daily doses of chasteberry doubled the rate of pregnancy. And while there were also a few additional herbs included in the testing compound, the researchers are convinced chasteberry brought about most of the results.

- In a study involving 52 women diagnosed with luteal phase defect, chasteberry resulted in not just a measurable increase in progesterone, but better hormone balance overall.

- In a double-blind placebo-controlled study of 30 women with fertility problems who took daily doses of chasteberry, 27 showed an increase in mid-cycle progesterone levels, and an increase in the number of pregnancies when compared to women who did not use this herb.

And that's just the beginning! Indeed, nearly every day we are discovering more about the powers of this beautiful little flower to impact female fertility in a big way.

My Personal Chasteberry Fertility Prescription: Since dosing is dependent on the type of problem you are trying to solve, how much you need to boost your fertility can be somewhat different for each woman.

That said, to increase fertility research published in the journal of the *American Family Physician* (AFP) suggests 4 mg per day of a standardized extract. In the United

---

Chasteberry Instead of Progresterone?

Q: *I've been diagnosed with a luteal phase defect and my doctor prescribed progesterone. Could I take Chasteberry instead?*

A: Chasteberry has, indeed, been proven in medical studies to be very helpful for the condition known as luteal phase defect - which simply means a lack of progesterone in the second half of the menstrual cycle. Check with your doctor first, but it's possible that chasteberry may work as well as progesterone, or certainly help increase it's effectiveness. Do not, however, take both together without your doctors's approval.

States, this formulation is available as Femaprin from Nature's Way – but other companies provide similar formulations. Just be sure to check the label to ensure you are getting a "standardized" formulation.

If you are using the fruit extract, which also comes packaged as a supplement (and the label would note that it is a fruit extract) then the AFP study recommends 20 to 40 mg per day, although higher doses (up to 1,800 mg per day) have been used with no safety issues or change in effectiveness noted. If your extract is fluid, this equals about 40 drops per day; if you are using a tincture then the dosing is 35 to 45 drops, three times daily.

You can use chasteberry in any form either continuously every day, or for just half of your cycle, beginning right after your menstrual bleed stops, and continuing through ovulation, and stopping within 24 hours afterwards. You would begin again at the start of the next cycle.

While chasteberry appears safe with no dramatic adverse reactions repoted, as with all natural compounds there is always a chance for side effects or even an occasional allergic reaction. Signs to look for include an increase in headaches, gastrointestinal difficulties, and lower abdominal complaints, and of course any typical signs of allergy including hives, itching, redness or swelling. If these

Fertility Booster # 2: Black Cohosh

Although best known as a "menopause" herb, what many women do not realize is the same kinds of hormonal upsets that cause hot flashes and night sweats in older women, can cause infertility in younger women. And therein lies the logic behind the use of black cohosh to boost fertility.

Also known as Actaea racemosa or sometimes as Cimicifuga racemosa – this flowering plant is native to North America and in fact it's first recorded use in the US was by Native Americans, who used it to treat many types of gynecologic disorders. Today, black cohosh has been the subject of over 20 clinical trials involving more than 3,000 women – all with great results!

Like other plants - including fruits and vegetables – black cohosh contains many different phytonutrients, including flavonoids and tannins . But the star player, in terms of fertility, appears to be a compound known as "triterpenoid glycosides " – which a number of key studies have shown does have mild estrogenic effects.

But more importantly, black cohosh has another property that allows it be so useful for both older and younger women : It is known as an "adaptogen". In herbal - speak this is an herb that can literally "adapt" to what your specific body needs are at the moment. So, for example, if your hormones are low and they need a boost, black cohosh can work on the pathways that increase production. If you are producing too much of one hormone and not enough of another, it can also help normalize levels. In this respect, Black Cohosh is almost the "perfect" fertility herb, working to help your body produce more of what you personally need to optimize hormone production. If you are under age 45 that can lead to increased fertility.

Moreover, there is also evidence that black cohosh has anti-spasmodic effects which can help prevent your newly fertilized egg from being pushed down your fallopian tube too quickly – resulting in an unhealthy implantation and an increased risk of miscarriage. By preventing these spasms, black cohosh can also be useful for women suffering from chronic miscarriage.

How To Use Black Cohosh To Get Pregnant

As helpful as this herb has proven to be, it's important to note that not all black cohosh is alike. Indeed, many experts believe that the success of this treatment is intimately tied to the specific black cohosh formulation you use – which in turn is tied to the level of active compounds it contains.

So, what should you take? To date, the vast majority of clinical trials conducted on black cohosh and yielding favorable results have all utilized a single brand of this herb: Remefemin. In fact, Remefemin has been the subject of over 90 scientific papers and has been tested on over 3,000 women suffering with low estrogen.

Not surprisingly, Remefemin is also the brand of black cohosh that is most often recommended by doctors, and I frequently recommend it as well.

My Personal Black Cohosh Fertility Prescription: In terms of dosing, the average amount needed to quell menopausal symptoms is between 40 mg and 80 mg per day. That said, to use this herb as a fertility enhancer I would recommend that you start with 40 mg daily and take it for at least 8 weeks before increasing the dosage.

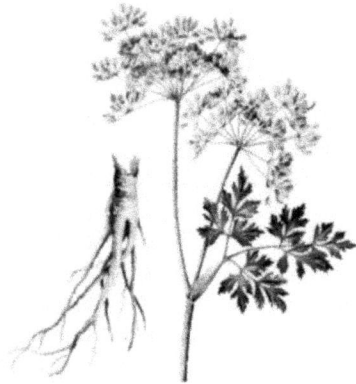

Fertility Booster # 3: Dong Quai

In the world of Chinese medicine, the herb known Dong Quai has been a mainstay of good health for thousands of years. In fact the root of Dong Quai is considered one of the most honored herbs in Chinese medicine, with a history of use that goes back more than 2,000 years.

As member of the celery family, it comes from the plant Angelica sinensis, and has been used to treat a variety of illnesses related to reproductive health including menstrual cramps, irregular cycles, and infrequent or absent periods, as well as taming symptoms of PMS.

But perhaps the most profound use of Dong Quai involves reducing the risk of recurrent miscarriage – a property frequently ascribed to this herbal treatment. Indeed, while it contains a number of important health compounds, among them is a natural chemical known as "coumadin" – which you may already know as the basis for the blood thinning drug of the same name.

And it is, in fact, the blood thinning properties of Dong Quai that may be responsible for its ability to reduce the risk of miscarriage.

Indeed, while any number of factors can be the cause of a pregnancy loss, one of the most common is the formation of tiny clots in the small blood vessels inside the uterus. When these develop, the nourishment from your body necessary to help your baby thrive and grow simply isn't delivered. Without it, your baby cannot survive – and so a miscarriage occurs. Dong Quai is believed to reduce this risk by helping to keep these tiny clots from forming.

Moreover, the coumadin found in Dong Quai also works as an anti-inflammatory which can be very helpful in reducing the presence of inflammatory compounds that might otherwise damage or even kill sperm before fertilization can take place. Additionally, another compound found in Dong Quai known as ferulic acid, can, when combined with the the coumadin compound, offers antispasmodic as well as muscle relaxing effects on your uterus. And this can further reduce your risk of miscarriage.

Because Dong Quai also has a toning effect on the muscles of the uterus, once you are pregnant you may find that you are better able to tolerate your pregnancy with fewer aches and pains. You may even have an easier delivery, all thanks to the pre-conception toning effects of Dong Quai!

My Personal Dong Quai Fertility Prescription – *with some precautions.*

The accepted dose of Dong Quai for women trying to get pregnant is three to four grams a day. Supplements of powdered Dong Quai root can be found in capsule form, as well as in tablets, tinctures and extracts. It can also be brewed as a tea.

Since Dong Quai has an extremely low toxicity profile, there is little chance that you can overdose or have a bad reaction.

That said, some side effects have been reported including a sensitivity to sunlight, particularly if you have fair skin. Dong Quai can also impact blood sugar and should not be used if you have diabetes or insulin resistance - or a related fertility condition such as PCOS.

If you have a very heavy menstrual cycle, or if you bleed excessively from fibroid tumors or polyps you should also not use Dong Quai. You should also stop this herb as soon as you believe you are pregnant.

You must also remain aware that Dong Quai can interact with a number of common prescription and over-the-counter medications including anti-inflammatory drugs, diuretics and some lithium based drugs used to treat bi polar disorder .

 It can also interfere with blood thinning medications such as Coumadin or Wafarin, or some medications for high blood pressure. If you are regularly using any of these medications check with your doctor before taking Dong Quai.

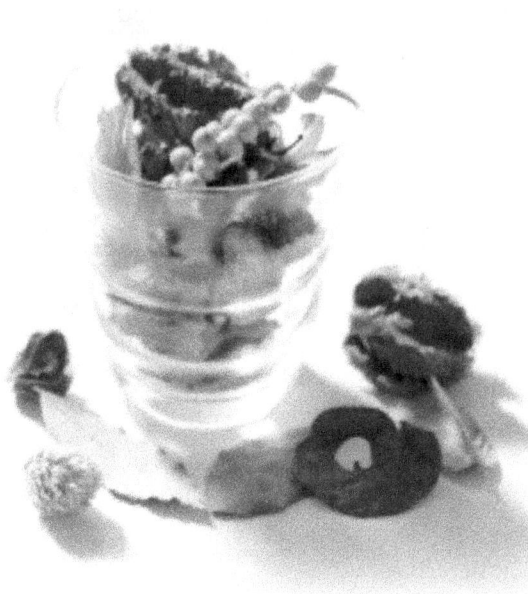

The Chinese Fertility Cocktail!

As helpful as I believe Dong Quai can be on its own, in traditional Chinese medicine (known as TCM) it is almost always prescribed as part of a group of herbs that work synergistically together, each one boosting the effect of the other.

For fertility, most Chinese medicine doctors prescribe a "fertility cocktail" consisting of a group of herbs – including Dong Quai – that work together to tone the uterus, improve hormone balance, reduce blood clotting and inflammation and generally improve the overall health of your reproductive system.

The herbs most often combined with Don Quai include Ligusticum, Rehmanii, and white peony – all of which are thought to work together in a way that promotes a healthy conception.

While there a number of companies offering this or a variation as a fertility supplement, if you are really serious about using Chinese medicine to improve your reproductive health, I would strongly suggest you seek out a Chinese medicine doctor who can customize your treatment based on your specific fertility needs. While most universities and teaching hospitals can refer you to a specialist in your area, you can also contact the American Association of Oriental Medicine (http://www.aaom.org/), or the National Certification **Commission for Acupuncture and Oriental Medicine** (NCCAOM) http://www.nccaom.org/ for a referral .

Fertility Booster # 4: Raspberry Leaf

One of the oldest herbs in recorded history, raspberry leaf has traditionally been used by women as far back as the bible as a uterine relaxant.

This herb not only reduces menstrual cramps and controls heavy bleeding *before you are pregnant*, the same anti-spasmodic effects may help reduce your risk of miscarriage after you conceive.

Some naturopathic doctors believe that when used prior to conception red raspberry leaf can encourage your newly fertilized egg to attach to your uterine lining and, most important, remain attached, again reducing the risk of miscarriage.

If you suffer with monthly bouts of PMS – or especially if you have been diagnosed with a luteal phase defect, (both problems characterized by a lack of progesterone) raspberry leaf extract can help. Indeed, in herbal circles this plant is actually known as a "phyto-progesterone" - a natural source of plant progesterone.

As a bonus, if you are trying to get pregnant during the hot summer months, Raspberry leaf can help bring liquids into your cells which in turn can help you avoid dehydration – a problem which can upset the balance of minerals in your body and temporarily impact your fertility.

Available in powdered form and sold as capsules, or in liquid form as a tincture, the usual supplement contains 400 mg per dose. Most herbalists recommend one to two capsules up to three times daily.

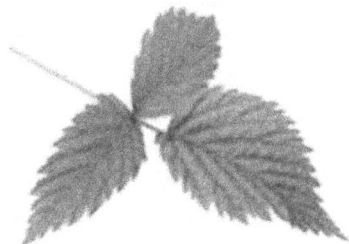

My Personal Raspberry Leaf Fertility Prescription: One of my favorite ways to "prescribe" raspberry leaf is via a freshly brewed tea made from the leaf. However, make certain that your tea actually contains *raspberry leaf* and not just raspberry flavoring or raspberry extract. You need the leaf, not the fruit to get the best results. Several cups per day should be sufficient to get the desire effect.

Fertility Booster # 5 : False Unicorn Root

With a long history of use within the Native American Indian community, false unicorn root is believed to encourage fertility by acting as a weak form of estrogen – helping to encourage ovulation in women with irregular cycles.

But much like black cohosh, this herb is also considered to be "adaptogenic" – meaning it can adjust its activity based on what your body needs at any given time. Often, the end result is both better hormone balance and more regular ovulation, along with the production of better and stronger eggs. This also helps reduce the risk of miscarriage.

My Personal False Unicorn Root Fertility Prescription: If you'd like to try this herb it is usually available as a liquid extract and the normal dosage is 1 teaspoon (or 6 to 8 drops) in a cup of water, two to three times daily. You can also use 1 to 2 grams of the root brewed into a pot of tea and it's safe to drink up to three cups per day. If you take the root tincture on its own, 1 teaspoon 3 times a day is the standard dosing.

One caution: For some women, anywhere from 5 to 15 drops of the extract or 3 to 4 cups of tea per day can cause nausea and vomiting. For this reason I recommend that you start slow with a small amount and gradually build your tolerance level. If you do begin to feel nauseous you'll automatically know your threshold – and know how much to cut back to relieve your symptoms.

Fertility Booster # 6: Red Clover

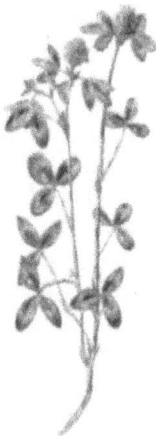

Although it's name sounds much like a weed you might be tempted to pull from your front garden, in reality Red Clover is actually a type of legume that comes from the same family as soybeans – and therein lies some of its power as a fertility herb.

Although it has gained a strong reputation as a hormone-balancing treatment used primarily to alleviate menopausal symptoms, these same effects can be equally important if you are a young woman suffering from a hormone imbalance.

Like soybeans, red clover derives its power from "isoflavones" – natural compounds with mild estrogenic effects. So why not just eat soybeans?

First, in addition to the two types of isoflavones found in soy - genisten and daidzen- red clover also contains biochannin A and formononetin, two more isoflavones believed to have greater hormone balancing properties.

But more importantly, unlike soy which has a decidedly "estrogenic" effect, red clover works as an adaptogen. So if your estrogen level is low Red Clover will increase it; if your level of estrogen is normal or even high, it can "down regulate" this hormone - meaning it keeps your body from experiencing an estrogen overload while still working to achieve a more normal hormonal balance overall. And this is something soy supplements cannot do.

Although red clover is technically classified as a legume, you can't eat it like a vegetable. You can however, purchase red clover teas, infusions or various dried products.

But if you're really serious about giving this compound a try, I would suggest you immediately look to red clover supplements. While there are a variety of different types to choose from, the most widely used brand – and the one tested in more clinical trials than any other – is Promensil. It is standardized to contain 40 mg of four key isoflavones , plus another weak plant estrogen known as coumasol, a compound similar to what is found in Dong Quai.

My Red Clover Fertility Prescription

The suggested amount for menopause symptoms is one 40 mg capsule of Promensil daily, with up to 2 capsules daily for severe symptoms.

I recommend that for re-balancing fertility hormones you stay with one capsule daily for 8 weeks, during which time you should monitor your cycle for regularity. You should also use various natural methods of monitoring your ovulation cycles (which you'll learn about later in this book).

I believe you will soon see positive signs in both areas – which is an indication that your fertility is blooming!

A few precautions: Red clover can interfere with the processing of some Medications so, if you are taking prescription or over-the-counter medications on a regular basis, (particularly if you are using Metformin with or without Clomid for the treatment of PCOS) talk to your doctor before taking this supplement since it has been known to lower blood sugar and may impact the effects of some drugs used to

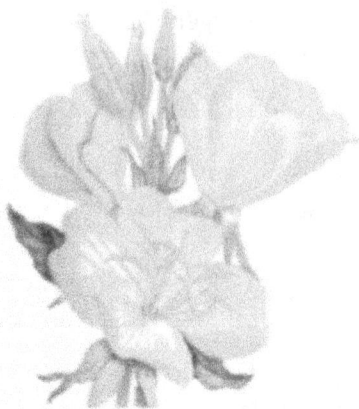

Fertility Booster # 7:
Evening Oil of Primrose

Derived from the small dark seeds of the Evening Primrose plant, the oil is rich in Vitamin E as well as as some essential fatty acids including linolenic acid (the same compound that is found in flax seed oil) and gamma linolenic acid also known as GLA. And therein may lie it's beneficial links to fertility.

Indeed, the key element in all these compounds is that they produce anti-inflammatory effects in the body. So, certainly if you have any inflammatory conditions linked to infertility – particularly endometriosis – Evening Oil of Primrose can help.

But perhaps more importantly, these same compounds also appear to have a regulating effect on certain key hormones related to conception. So, it would appear that Evening Oil of Primrose might also be helpful when a hormone imbalance is keeping you from getting pregnant.

While a number of important studies have shown that Evening Oil of Primrose works well as a treatment for symptoms of PMS , not everyone agrees. Indeed, at least one meta-analysis of the studies on Evening Oil of Primrose revealed flaws in many of the trails, with some of the most convincing effects of this compound unable to be duplicated in subsequent studies.

That said, it is my personal belief - backed up by my professional experience - that this compound can help you. This is true not only if you have PMS, but also if you suffer a similar hormonal imbalance linked to infertility – particularly since we know that essential fatty acids are such key players in many areas of reproductive health.

In addition, there also appears to be some evidence - though this time largely anecdotal - that Evening Oil of Primrose may help thin cervical mucus, making it more "sperm friendly." While there is no true scientific evidence to show this is true, there are isolated reports from women who say that it does help. So again, if you find that your cervical mucus production is low, or that it is very sticky and thick, you might want to give Evening Oil of Primrose a try.

My Evening Oil of Primrose Fertility Prescription:

1500mg - 3,000 mg daily – taken in 500 mg doses spread throughout the day.

Evening Oil of Primrose and PMS

Q: *Will Evening Oil of Primrose help my PMS symptoms - and will that help me get pregnant?*

A: There are some studies to show that Evening Oil of Primrose can be helpful for some women who suffer with symptoms of PMS. Others show the advantages are small, if any.

That said I have personally seen many women feel much better taking this supplement and I believe it can help.

If you are having problems getting pregnant that you believe are related to a hormone imbalance - which is very common - then yes, Evening Oil of Primrose could help to increase your chance of getting pregnant.

While this compound has an excellent safety profile it should not be used during pregnancy, or during the second half of the menstrual cycle if you are trying to conceive (See precautions below).

Some Important Precautions: The best time to use this supplement is daily, right after your period ends, and stopping mid-cycle as soon as you ovulate. This is important since there are some isolated reports that Evening Oil of Primrose may increase uterine contractions. As such, if you do conceive, the contractions related to Evening Oil of Primrose could rush your embryo down your fallopian too quickly (before your uterus is fully prepared for implantation). If your fertilized egg does reach your uterus in the correct amount of time, these same contractions might prevent it from properly adhering to the uterine wall.

You can however, safely use either omega 3 fatty acid supplements or Flax Seed Oil supplements during the second half of your cycle to help continue the anti-inflammatory and other positive effects of essential fatty acids.

In addition, do not use Evening Oil of Primrose prior to surgery, (even fertility procedures) or if you are at risk for seizures. Do not use this supplement if you are taking phenothiazine-related medications, anti-platelet drugs, thrombolytics, low-molecular-weight heparins, or anticoagulant drugs. It's also important to point out that The German Commission E has not approved the use of Evening Oil of Primrose for any specific purpose.

Fertility Booster # 8: DHEA

Although not an herb, a new natural treatment known as DHEA (short for **Dehydroepiandrosterone**) is fast proving to be as effective as many herbal supplements –and for many women far exceed that which any herb can accomplish.

But what is this supplement and how does it work?

DHEA is a precursor compound that the body uses to make steroid hormones, including some that are directly involved in reproduction. Moreover, many fertility experts are now turning to DHEA supplements to help increase egg production, as well as egg quality in women having problems getting pregnant. For some, the effect has proven to be so strong they were able to achieve a natural pregnancy – even after IVF treatments failed!

According to New York fertility experts Dr. Norbert Gleicher and Dr. David Barad, who have conducted studies on DHEA, it works by increasing production and metabolism of steroid hormones including estrogens and androgens.

It also appears to increase certain other compounds related to egg development, thus providing a kind of overall boost to fertility – particularly for those women over age 40 who may be having difficulty producing eggs. Which was precisely the age group on which Dr. Barad's studies were conducted.

Over the course of his two year research, Dr. Barad used DHEA in the treatment of 120 IVF patients all over the age of 40 , most of whom had been told by other fertility experts that donor eggs were their only option for getting pregnant.

After treatment with DHEA, Dr. Barad observed a marked increase in natural egg production and quality in all of the women, as well as an increase in pregnancy rates, when compared to women who did not take the DHEA supplements. Of those 120 women in the study, to date, over two dozen were able to get pregnant using DHEA supplements in conjuction with traditional IVF procedures using their own eggs.

His studies have also shown that DHEA improves IVF pregnancy rates, and decreases the rate of miscarriage, as well as increasing the rate of natural pregnancy in couples who are having problems conceiving.

> ## More Is Not Better!
>
> As helpful as DHEA can be to some women, remain aware that it is, essentially, a male hormone, so you need only very small amounts to see a result.

Dr. Gleicher reminds us that of the women in their studies who used DHEA supplements most reported feeling better and stronger overall, with improved memory and cognitive function and an increase in their sex drive.

So, can DHEA help increase your fertility? Although the studies were conducted on women who were involved in IVF treatments, still if you are over age 35 and having problems getting pregnant naturally, it is certainly worth giving DHEA a try.

As to whether or not it can encourage fertility in younger women, we can't say for certain but if you are having problems getting pregnant, and particularly if you are over age 35, then it certainly might be worth giving DHEA supplements a try.

Of course, if you know you are ovulating regularly, and your egg production is already good, this is probably not the right supplement for you.

Also be aware that because DHEA is essentially a male hormone, you only need very small amounts to see a result. In fact, using larger amounts, while not necessarily dangerous, will result in some unpleasant side effects, including oily skin and hair, and acne.

My DHEA Fertility Prescription:

The dosage of DHEA used in the fertility studies was 25 mg, three times a day.

If you are not certain if you are ovulating, or you are under age 35 I would suggest you begin with 25 mg twice a day, and add more if needed. If you are over age 35, then 25 mg three times a day would likely help you.

When purchasing a DHEA supplement, it's important that you seek out a compounding pharmacy, which makes products from scratch. They can help ensure that you are getting a top quality DHEA supplement with the proper potency.

If you are unable to find a compounding pharmacy in your area, several experts who have done clinical testing on DHEA recommend the website www.DHEA.com as a source for high quality, pharmaceutical grade supplements.

The Herbs That Help Male Fertility

While there are a variety of herbs that have been associated with male fertility, there is little in the way of medical studies showing they work. Of course this doesn't mean they don't – it just means that we don't yet have the scientific proof to back up what can sometimes be generations or even centuries of successful use.

So with this in mind, what follows are the herbs that are most commonly associated with an increase in male fertility. While a few have been proven out in medical studies, others have strong cultural associations as well as credible anecdotal support.

Remember, it's important for your partner to also choose a high quality supplement from a credible and well known company. Again, this is important to insure that the product is pure and processed correctly and free of contaminants, particularly pesticides, which can be harmful to his fertility.

He should also follow the directions from the company, on how much to use and remember that when it comes to herbal products, more is not always better. In fact sometimes taking too much of a substance can cause an effect opposite of what you are trying to achieve.

So your partner should not deviate too far from the recommended amounts on each product.

Also, it's best to try each of these supplements separately before attempting to combine them – and certainly they should never be taken all at once. By testing out each herb separately for 8 to 12 weeks, it's much easier to judge which are the most personally effective.

- ## Panax Ginseng

  For centuries this has been known as the " male tonic", used by generations of Chinese medicine practitioners as a way to improve overall male health. Now studies show it may have a direct impact on testosterone, increasing levels of this hormone as well as increasing sperm count. Siberian ginseng (*Eleutherococcus senticosus*) has also been shown to be similarly helpful.

- ## Astragalus (*Astragalus membranaceus*)

  According to a study published in the journal *Alternative Medicine Review*, researchers tested the extracts of 18 major Chinese medicinal plants for their ability to increase sperm motility. Of the 18, only Astragalus was shown to significantly increase the swimming ability of sperm by some 22%. While this was an in vitro test wherein the extracts were directly added to the sperm, still, many believe that when taken internally as an herbal extract, the effects on sperm will be similar.

- ## Saw palmetto (*Serenoa repens*)

  This herb first came to prominence as a treatment for benign prostate disease. Now, however, it is quickly gaining a reputation as an overall tonic for the male reproductive system and may have some positive effects on healthy sperm production.

- ## Maca Root

  This powerful plant contains a full complement of amino acids, complex carbohydrates, vitamins B1, B2, C, E and the minerals calcium, phosphorous, zinc, magnesium and iron. As such, it has been used by many South American cultures for generations as a way to increase the production of testosterone, encourage the production of healthy sperm, and generally tone up the male reproductive system – even to the point of increasing libido in some men.

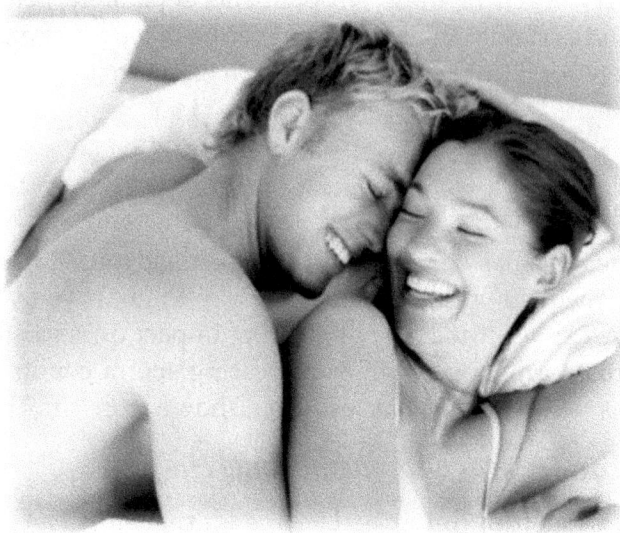

Natural Treatments
For You & Your Partner

While the vitamins mentioned in the previous chapter, and the herbs you read about in this chapter make up the largest share of natural fertility boosters, there are, in fact, a number of other supplements that, while they fall outside these categories, have been shown to help.

Some are derived from foods – and actually considered dietary supplements – others are a blend of nutrients and herbs that have been shown to work synergistically to enhance fertility and improve the reproductive profile of both men and women.

What follows are my choices for the most important of these supplements – and the ones that have the most clinical research backing. Many are also the supplements I have found to be helpful for my patients.

As with other supplements mentioned in this and previous chapters, remember, however, that results do take time. So, have patience and keep a positive outlook , and I'm quite certain you will benefit from at least one of these formulations.

Boost Your Fertility With Omega 3's !

As you read in an earlier chapter, omega 3's are a group of essential fatty acids that can have a profound impact on your fertility. The two omega 3 compounds most useful to fertility are called EPA (Eicosapentaenoic acid) and DHA (docosahexaenoic acid). Found primarily in fish oil, among their many benefits is countering the fertility-robbing effects of insulin resistance, and if you are diagnosed with PCOS or another ovulatory -related problem, these fatty acids can be particularly helpful.

In one study researchers found that simply adding more omega 3 fatty acids to the diet worked to kick-start ovulation even in women who were not ovulating at all. There is also evidence to show that the anti-inflammatory effects of omega 3 fatty acids can also help to re-balance hormones and increase blood flow to the uterus, which in turn can help foster a healthy implantation.

But it's not just women who benefit from omega 3's! In men, omega 3 fatty acids are found in very high concentrations in the tails of healthy sperm - plus they work as hormone regulators, helping to tone the male reproductive system overall.

In fact, this nutrient is so important to male fertility in one study recently published in *the Journal of Lipids* doctors found that an ample supply of omega 3 fatty acids in the diet could actually reverse some forms of male infertility related to sperm abnormalities. Moreover, when levels of this nutrient drop, there may be a decrease in the number of healthy sperm available for fertilization. Studies also show that in men with a low supply of omega 3 fatty acids, sperm contain more cholesterol - which slows down the rate of maturity and affects sperm motility, all of which can lead to infertility.

Why You Both Need Omega 3 Supplements

Although these fatty acid compounds are considered "essential" to both male and female health as well as fertility, oddly enough your body is unable to make omega 3 fatty acids on its own. Indeed, they must be derived from your diet. And while I have always believed that dietary sources and natural foods are among the best ways to consume this nutrient (see Chapter Three for more information on the foods highest in Omega 3) I have also found that even among those couples who have a "good" diet, omega 3 fatty acid consumption still frequently comes up short. For this reason – and because this nutrient is so important to your overall health and your fertility – I also frequently recommend supplementation.

Although there are many types of Omega 3 fatty acid supplements, most experts agree that those which come from cold water fish such as salmon, mackerel, and hoki, (a New Zealand fish) are among the best.

That said, it's important to note that not all fish oils – even from these fish - are created equal!

This is particularly true when it comes to issues like mercury contamination. Indeed, one reason I have found that so many of my patients were not eating more fish was because of fears and worries over contamination from mercury and other potentially harmful chemicals.

The good news: There *are* fish oil supplements that are safe – in some instances much safer than eating fish.

So, how do you find the ones that will help without doing harm?

Read the product label and look for the words "molecularly distilled". This is a process that uses high heat to remove all toxins from the fish oil - and in the process also removes that "fishy" aftertaste that can repeat on some people.

While there are some product manufacturers who claim that molecular distillation also removes some of the potency of the fish oil (mostly by changing the original ratio of all the nutrients found naturally in fish) when it comes to fertility I believe molecular distillation can be helpful, particularly since some of the chemicals contaminants found in unprocessed fish oil have been linked to reproductive problems.

My personal opinion is that it's better to have a fish oil supplement that is slightly less powerful, but clean in terms of contaminants that can impact fertility. If need be you can always increase your dosage to get more benefits.

And again, don't forget that you also have the option of seeking out supplements made from fish that swim in pristine clean waters. As mentioned earlier, these include hoki fish from protected waters off the coast of New Zealand as well as salmon from the pristine clean waters off the coast of Scandinavia.

While these fish generally are not subjected to the harmful chemical pollutants found in other parts of the world, some of these supplements can also be very costly, so if you're on a tight budget this might not be an option for you.

My Personal Omega 3 Prescription for Male & Female Fertility:

Between 800 - 1000 mg or 1 gram of EPA and DHA daily. This usually translates to one to two capsules a day depending on the strength.

The best products will be those containing a minimum of 180 mg of EPA and 120 mg of DHA in conjunction with other fatty acids so you get a good balance without sacrificing the therapeutic levels necessary to see results.

Precaution: According to the FDA you can safely take up to 3,000 mg (or 3 grams) daily with no adverse effects, but I definitely would *not* go above that amount without talking to your doctor first.

In fact, because this supplement can have blood thinning effects, you and your partner should definitely check with your doctors before taking this supplement in any amount.

The Fish Oil Alternative Supplement

If you want to avoid fish oil , but still want the benefits of Omega 3 fatty acids, seek out supplements made from flax seed oil.

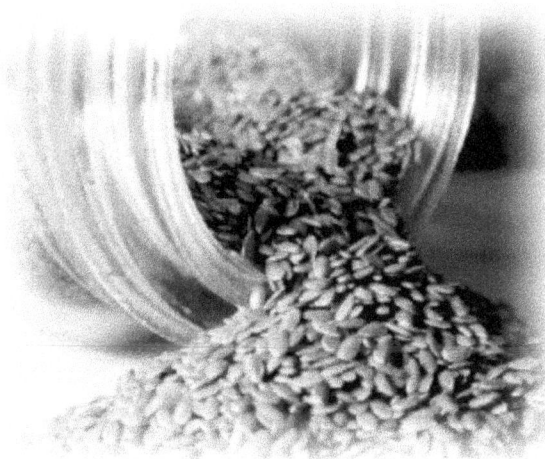

While you won't be getting either EPA or DHA directly, what you will get is a compound known as ALA (alpha linolenic acid) which the body converts into the same compounds you would get if if you took omega 3 fatty acids directly.

Another option is walnut seed oil supplements, which also contain the same ALA compounds as flax.

Although neither flax seed or walnut supplements are quite as powerful as taking fish oil supplements, still they can prove helpful if fish oil is something you just can't tolerate. It also does not leave you with the same "fishy" after-taste or gastric issues that some types of fish supplements cause.

If you do choose either a flax seed supplement or a walnut oil supplement look for products that contain at least 1000 mg of the *seed oil,* containing at least 500 mg of alpha linolenic acid, 110 mg of linoleic acid and 110 mg of oleic acid. These numbers – or those close to them – should be on the label.

If your supplement contains approximately these levels, I recommend that you take two per day, with meals.

The Fertility Nutrient: CoQ10

Because it's so often mentioned in the same context as vitamins, many people believe that the nutrient known as CoQ10 is in fact a vitamin.

But in truth it's really a compound that is produced naturally by every living cell in the body. It is necessary for the production of another compound known as ATP (adenosine triphosphate) which is actually the "fuel" of all living cells.

Without adequate C0Q10 , ATP supply dwindles – and that means cells won't get the nutrients they need to thrive - including the cells involved in egg production and maturation in women and sperm maturation in men.

Moreover, CoQ10 is also a powerful antioxidant, which can also give both you and your partner a natural fertility boost.

In terms of specific effects on fertility, studies have shown that directly following miscarriage, levels of CoQ10 are exceedingly low - a fact which has led to some serious speculation concerning the role of CoQ10 in preventing miscarriage.

While we have no definitive studies showing that this is the case, there is certainly enough scientific suggestion - along with some clear cut evidence on the antioxidant powers of COQ10 - to recommend it as a fertility supplement for women.

Moreover, in men, CoQ10 is present in large amounts in seminal fluid - the substance which carries sperm from your partner's body into your body. As such, research indicates CoQ10 helps energize sperm, increasing their ability to swim through your reproductive system and reach your egg.

There is also research showing fertilization rates rise when Coenzyme Q10 supplements are given to men undergoing the male fertility procedure known as ICSI.

My Fertility Prescription for C0Q10 : 60 mg – 100 mg capsules, once daily for women; 200 mg daily for men.

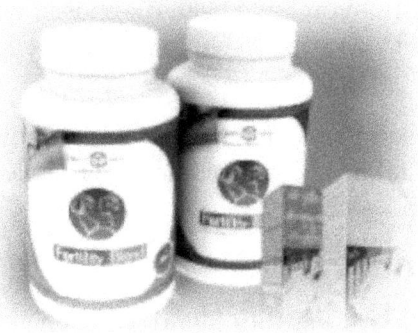

Fertility Blend & Other Support Supplements:
What You Must Know

Whether you and your partner are just thinking about getting pregnant – or if you've already been trying for quite some time - you have no doubt heard about a number of supplements being sold specifically as "fertility boosters", with formulations specific to both men and women.

While most contain the same nutrients, herbs and compounds you've already read about in this chapter still, many companies claim that their particular way of combining these ingredients contributes to the success of their products.

While this may be true, to date, only one of these supplements has undergone testing within the fertility medicine arena – and I'm happy to say it did appear to have at least some impact on getting pregnant. That supplement is known as *Fertility Blend.*

Currently it is available in two formulas – one for men, one for women. The female formula contains a proprietary blend of amino acids, herbs, vitamins and minerals including chasteberry, green tea, vitamin E, selenium, folic acid, vitamins B 6, B 12, iron, zinc and magnesium, and the amino acid L arginine.

The male version contains a combination of the amino acid L-carnitine, along with Vitamins C and E, green tea, selenium, ferulic acid (found in Dong Quai) , as well as zinc, and vitamins B6, B12 and folate (folic acid).

While the female version has undergone rigorous gold-standard double-blind placebo controlled studies, the male version has not been subjected to the same level of testing. Still, promising results are seen with the use of both formulations.

In one small but significant double blinded study conducted at Stamford University, doctors tested Fertility Blend on 93 women age 24 to 42, all of whom had been unsuccessful in getting pregnant for a minimum of at least 6 months. After taking the supplement once daily for 3 months, the researchers noted an increase in progesterone production, along with an increase in the number of days with an elevated BBT (basal body temperature) in the second half of the menstrual cycle – indicating an important increase in hormonal production has occurred.

As such this formulation may be especially useful if you have been diagnosed with a fertility problem known as "luteal phase defect", a problem characterized by low progesterone in the second half of your cycle.

Perhaps most important, Fertility Blend increased pregnancy rates. According to the Stamford study, some 32% of the women taking Fertility Blend were able to conceive, while just 10% conceived in the placebo group.

Will Fertility Blend Help You and Your Partner?

Right about now you may be asking yourself why, if Fertility Blend has such good results, should I even bother taking any of the individual herbs, minerals or vitamins discussed in these last few chapters ?

Well the truth is, Fertility Blend does contains a great many of the individual nutrients I have recommended thus far. So in this respect I would say that taking this supplement might indeed be a good place to start your experimentation with natural fertility formulations.

That said, it's also important to remember that every person's body is slightly different – which also means that what it takes to encourage fertility in you or your partner, can be slightly different as well. Your individual body chemistry, your weight, your diet and your nutrient status, even your overall health are all factors which not only influence your fertility, but also the effectiveness of any treatment you take.

So, while for some a product like Fertility Blend might be the perfect answer, for others, experimenting with the individual herbs mentioned in this chapter and the vitamins mentioned in the previous chapter may be more beneficial. Indeed, while the 32% pregnancy rate of Fertility Blend is impressive, it's wise to remember that 68 % of the women taking this supplement *did not get pregnant.* This doesn't mean that the formulation failed– or that the women failed. It only means that for these women perhaps a slightly different configuration of natural ingredients might have been necessary to enhance their individual fertility profile.

As such, if you and your partner try a product like Fertility Blend and it does not yield the results you're looking for, don't be afraid to look to some of the individual supplements and vitamins I have recommended. You can either take these in addition to the Fertility Blend supplement, or replace it completely with your own customized formulation.

Either way the end result can be a blend of ingredients that are best suited to enhance your personal fertility profile and help you get pregnant.

Choosing Fertility Supplements: A Few Final Words

Whether you're shopping in your local pharmacy, or, as most couples do today, online, you have no doubt already seen that in addition to Fertility Blend there are many more pre-packaged fertility supplements on the market. Many claim they are "Doctor Approved", or they boast that they have been "shown in testing" to work.

What's key to remember however, is that unless the company can provide references to medical studies – and hopefully publication of those studies in bona fide medical journals - claims made by the products may be just that ... claims, and nothing more.

Does this mean they won't be effective or help you ?   No, it does not mean that. Some of these products may work as well as Fertility Blend, some may work better – and others may not work at all.

So how can you tell which ones are worth trying?

In terms of individual results, *you really can't tell until you give them a try*. However, you can narrow your chances of getting a more effective product if you look for the following information associated with each treatment:

- Standardization: All herbs used in the product should be "Standardized" to contain the exact amount of the effective ingredients it says it contains.

- Effective Levels of Nutrients: Using my suggested supplement recommendations as a guide you should read product labels to see if the blended formulations contain enough of the key ingredient to make a difference. If for example I am suggesting 60 mg of a particular herb and the blend contains just 5 mg, it's doubtful you will get the desired effect.

- Choose products with a minimal amount of fillers, binders, artificial ingredients or preservatives.

- When possible look for herbal ingredients harvested from organic crops.

- Avoid products with too many ingredients. If a fertility supplement label starts to look like a recipe for vegetable soup, then it's doubtful that any one ingredient will be represented in a large enough dose to have an impact on your fertility.

Moreover, while it's true that the herbs and other nutrients mentioned in this chapter are natural products, it's important to remember that they must be taken in balance , since too much of any one thing could harm you. Indeed, when it comes to enhancing fertility *more is not always better* – so remember not to take everything you hear about all at the same time!

Certainly maintaining a healthy diet, one that is high in fruits, vegetables, fiber and lean proteins, should always be your foundation – along with a high potency vitamin-mineral supplement.

From here you can add any of the herbal or other suggested supplements – but do so with some selectivity in mind.

You can try a few compounds simultaneously, but don't try to take the whole shopping cart at once! If you watch your body, and more importantly, *listen to your body* – you will begin to know instinctively which of these compounds are helping you to feel better, normalizing your menstrual cycles, encouraging regular ovulation, and ultimately optimizing your personal fertility profile so you can get pregnant fast.

Likewise, if either of you take a product and don't feel well, or if you see negative effects on your menstrual cycle or symptoms of PMS or if your partner experiences smaller ejaculations or develops potency problems, then reduce the dosage or stop taking the supplement altogether. I have always believed that our bodies instinctively know when something is right for us. And if you tune in to this "natural health frequency" you'll soon learn to decipher your body's signals as well. In fact, some of you may remember one of my earliest books was titled *"Listen To Your Body"* and I called it that for a reason - because I know that when you do listen and pay attention to your body, you can achieve your personal best – and your best health. And that's the first step to making a healthy baby!

Chapter Six

Fitness & Fertility:

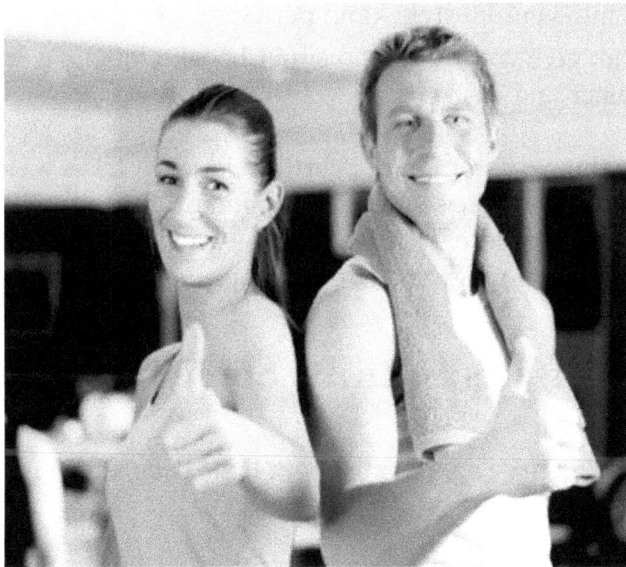

Getting Your Body Ready For Conception

O ver the past decade, and particularly over the last several years, the words "Diet and Exercise" have taken center-stage in the health news arena.

Protection from heart disease, high blood pressure, diabetes and even cancer, have all been linked to exercise and weight control, which are now seen as paramount to living a healthier and longer life.

Although we have heard less about the impact of these factors on fertility, I can assure you that there is no shortage of research in this area. Indeed, every day we continue to learn more about the increasingly important role that weight control and exercise can play in optimizing fertility, in both men and women.

And the really good news is that very small changes in either area can yield huge results. For example, for some men and women losing – or gaining – as little as 10 pounds can boost chances of getting pregnant by a whopping 50%!

For others, an activity as simple as walking 3 times a week can have an equally dramatic impact on fertility. In fact, by incorporating just a few simple weight and fitness guidelines into your lifestyle – and perhaps making a few very small changes - I promise you can give your fertility a super boost, while maximizing your ability to get pregnant faster and easier.

For these reasons, the next stop on our fertility journey takes a closer look at how weight management and exercise can come together to impact your fertility – and more importantly, the simple, easy ways that you and your partner can optimize not just your chance of getting pregnant, but also improve your overall health.

How Weight Affects Fertility: Some Important News

First and foremost, when we are talking about links between weight and fertility it's important for you to know two things.

- The first is that it's not just excess weight that can impact fertility. Indeed, being underweight can sometimes have an even greater impact on getting pregnant than being overweight.

- The second thing is that weight issues are not just a woman's fertility problem. Male fertility is also sensitive to weight gain and loss, affecting everything from hormonal output to sperm production.

That said, the exact ways in which weight impacts fertility can take some very different routes – depending on whether you or your partner need to lose – or gain – a few pounds. And by the way, I also want to reiterate again that it doesn't take a very big shift in weight to make a very big difference in your fertility. As I mentioned earlier, I have seen many couples go from infertile to fertile by simply losing or gaining as

---

little as 10 pounds in 6 weeks or less. So, the "investment" in your fertility future is really minimal compared to the enormous return your efforts will bring.

But how exactly does weight impact fertility – and what kinds of problems can it cause? When it comes to female fertility, among the theories quickly proving true involve links between fat cells – medically known as "adipocytes" - and hormone production, particularly estrogen, which you already know is the basis for all egg production.

While most of the estrogen necessary for conception is manufactured by your ovaries, what you may not know is that fat cells *also produce estrogen*. So, the more fat cells you have, the more estrogen your body produces. Conversely, the fewer fat cells you have, the less overall estrogen you have circulating through your bloodstream.

Because it is critical to your reproductive biochemistry to maintain this hormone at a specific level during various times of your monthly fertility cycle, whenever estrogen levels fall too much outside the norm – either too high or too low – problems can occur. This is true whether your estrogen levels are being impacted by a problem within your ovaries, or because of too few or two many fat cells. Either way, the end result can affect egg production and release, as well as put your monthly menstrual cycle into a tailspin!

How does this happen?

As you read earlier, in order for your ovaries to begin manufacturing and releasing eggs, your brain must produce a hormone known as FSH (follicle stimulating hormone). Simply put, FSH tells your ovaries to start processing your egg follicles into actual eggs. What's key, however, is that FSH gets its signal from estrogen. So, when estrogen levels are low, as they are at the conclusion of each month's menstrual bleeding, it signals the brain that it's time for a new cycle to begin. As such, FSH kicks in and starts the process rolling.

But what happens when, due to an increased number of fat cells, you have an excess of estrogen in your bloodstream? Your brain responds by thinking you don't need any FSH stimulation – so production of this hormone is turned off. When this occurs, your ovaries don't receive the "egg making" message at all – and suddenly the entire ovulation/reproductive cycle is disrupted. In fact, many women who are overweight frequently report irregular cycles, caused, at least in part, by a lack of FSH stimulation.

But it's not just irregular cycles that can occur. Women who are overweight often have a much more difficult time getting pregnant – with the amount of extra weight frequently correlating to the level of difficulty conceiving. Indeed, in one Dutch study of some 3,000 women, doctors found for every extra unit of body mass or BMI (a measurement of total body fat) there is a 4% drop in the chance of getting pregnant. Writing in the journal *Human Reproduction*, the researchers suggest that the more overweight a woman is, the more likely she is to have problems getting pregnant.

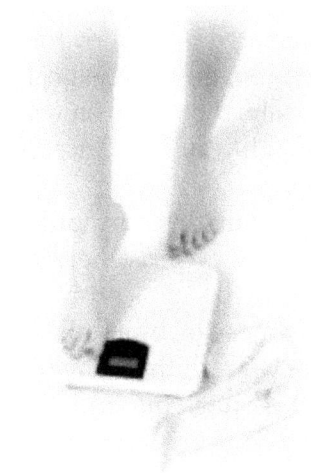

Too Skinny To Get Pregnant?

Once upon a time having a "model figure" meant you were curvy in "all the right places" - including your hips. Not coincidentally, these same "curves" also represented "fertility" - and are what made a woman very attractive to a man, both on a visual and hormonal level. Indeed, studies have revealed that men are frequently attracted – on an unconscious hormonally driven level – to women that they view as "fertile". And part of that fertility picture is the classic "Goddess" curvy body.

Today, however, our definition of "model perfect" has changed. In fact, in many areas of the world being extremely underweight is now considered the "ideal" body type – and one we have come to culturally worship and even idolize.

Unfortunately, however, this is a very dangerous ideal   -   dangerous not only for your overall health, but in particular for your fertility. Why? Simply put, you can be too skinny to get pregnant.

While we often associate weight-fertility problems with carrying too many pounds, the truth is that when a woman is too thin, just as many fertility problems can occur.

In fact, doctors have long known that women who have almost no body fat – such as marathon runners or professional dancers - are frequently diagnosed with annovulation, a condition where no eggs are being made or ovulated. Certainly in my professional experience I have found this to be true time and again. Many times my office was packed with models, athletes and dancers in a panic because their menstrual cycle had completely shut down. Some of them even believed they were pregnant, because their period had stopped. You can just imagine the surprise and even shock when I told that no, they weren't pregnant – and that if they didn't gain a few pounds they might never be able to have a baby.

Indeed studies show that complete hormonal shutdown can occur if your body fat dips just 10 to 15 percent below the normal 29% (a BMI of around 25). In fact, even just a slight drop below normal to a body fat level of 22% (a BMI of 19 to 20), can disrupt hormonal production enough to make it more difficult to get pregnant.

But why does this happen? As you read earlier, the brain chemicals necessary to kick-start the egg making process can be influenced by body fat. But it's not just a high level of body fat that can throw this chemistry into a tailspin. It can also happen when you don't have *enough* body fat.

Indeed when body fat levels drop too low, it sends a signal to your brain that your body is not adequately prepared to nourish a new life. And that in turn begins to disrupt all the brain circuitry involved in initiating a reproductive cycle. Depending on the degree to which this disruption occurs, any number of problems can result, including a sharp decline in egg production and release.

But even if ovulation does occur, and your egg becomes fertilized, being underweight dampens the production of hormones necessary to build a strong uterine lining. Without this, your fertilized egg may fail to attach to your uterus and grow. This is one reason why very thin women are at greater risk for early miscarriage.

Ultimately, if you remain severely underweight for a significant period of time, your menstrual cycle may stop completely, making it impossible to get pregnant. While most often this can be changed by simply restoring your body to a normal weight, if left to go on long enough, permanent infertility can sometimes result.

Hormones, Weight and Female Fertility:
An Important New Discovery

While we have long known that weight impacts fertility, only recently has research given us a clue as to exactly why this occurs. The basis of this new research revolves around a relatively new hormone know as "leptin ". 'From the Greek word Leptos – which actually means "thin" - leptin is a protein hormone that is produced by fat tissue. In fact, you may have already heard about leptin (as well as another newly discovered hormone known as ghrelin) in relation to studies on weight loss. Here doctors learned that fluctuations in both leptin and ghrelin can influence not only weight gain and loss, but also how well our metabolism works. And here is where the interesting link to fertility also came to light.

In studies conducted at both Brown University in Rhode Island and Harvard Medical School in Massachusetts doctors discovered that once leptin leaves your fat cells it travels through your blood stream to an area of your brain known as the hypothalamus. You may remember from an earlier chapter this is "hormone central" – the area of your brain that secretes chemicals that put the entire egg production and ovulation process in motion.

More specifically the researchers discovered that when leptin arrives in the hypothalamus, it acts like a switch, turning on a chemical chain reaction that stimulates first your pituitary gland, then your thyroid. This in turn sends out a body-wide message to increase energy production necessary for a wide variety of bodily functions, including not only calorie burning, but also reproduction.

But what happens when body fat is too low? Not enough leptin is produced. And this in turn signals the hypothalamus that there is an energy crisis. To conserve energy the hypothalamus responds by shutting down all "non-essential" body functions. One of the first of those functions to go: Reproduction. Indeed, there is now research documenting that when leptin levels drop low enough, the brain fails to produce either FSH or LH – so egg production and ovulation are unable to occur.

Although it seems that only thin women would be affected by a snafu in leptin production, women who are overweight are also affected. Why?

When the brain is continually bombarded with an oversupply of leptin – as it is when we have *too many* fat cells - it becomes desensitized to its effects, and begins to act almost as if no leptin is being produced at all! The end result: You gain even more weight, you produce even more leptin, and it becomes increasingly harder to get pregnant.

Additionally, it's important to note that the ability to produce leptin in the proper amounts is also ruled somewhat by genetics. If your leptin gene is defected – which is sometimes the case for those who suffer with extreme obesity - you will also suffer with a type of a weight-related infertility, even if your level of body fat is normal. As such, if you are at a good weight and no other cause for your fertility problems can be found, it's important to get a genetic test for the leptin gene.

Weight and Male Fertility:
What Your Partner Must Know

Because male fertility – and the production of sperm – is also dependent upon a finely tuned network of balanced hormone production, your partner's weight can also play a key role in helping to optimize *his* fertility and ultimately influence *your* chances of conception. In fact, in much the same way those fat cells within *your* body produce estrogen, so too do the fat cells in a man's body produce estrogen.

While it's normal for men to have small amounts of this hormone circulating through their body, when estrogen levels go too high – to the point where they dominate testosterone levels - his sperm production and his fertility can be dramatically compromised.

How much can he be affected by excess weight? In one study of some 1500 couples struggling with infertility conducted by the US National Institutes of Health, researchers discovered that being just 20 pounds overweight increases a man's risk of being infertile by about 10%.

In fact, the study also found that a man's BMI – or body mass index – (a way to record fat levels) was actually an independent risk factor for infertility. And this held true even after adjusting for other confounding factors such as a smoking, alcohol intake or chemical exposures.

Moreover they also found that the more a man weighs, the greater his risk of infertility.

More recent studies have shown that men who are obese have lower semen quality in general, as well as hormonal issues that might contribute to fertility problems.

So while we know that weight impacts a man's fertility, what we are less sure of is which comes first: The weight gain or the hormonal decline leading to infertility.

Indeed, while we know that gaining weight can dampen the production of testosterone, more recently we found out that in some men, a drop in testosterone precipitates weight gain.

In these men, some biochemical snafu causes a decline in testosterone, which in turn creates a number of metabolic changes, at least some of which lead to weight gain. The excess weight drives testosterone levels down even further, thus setting up a vicious cycle of metabolic imbalance that ultimately affects not just a man's fertility but his overall health.

While any number of factors can cause testosterone levels to decline, among middle aged men and older, the drop is usually part of the natural aging process. That said, younger men are not off the hook. Stress, chemical exposures, smoking, and alcohol consumption can reduce testosterone levels as well, even in young men, thus making it harder for them to control their weight – and their fertility.

But regardless of which comes first – the drop in testosterone or the weight gain - what we do know is that losing weight and getting your BMI as close to normal as possible will definitely give a natural boost to sperm production and fertility.

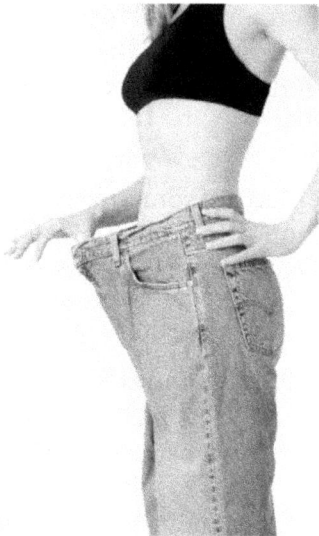

Belly Fat : Why It's Especially Bad For Male & Female Fertility

Although an excess of fat cells located anywhere in the body can impact the finely tuned hormonal network necessary for conception, recent research has shown gaining weight in one particular area of the body can be especially harmful. That area, is the belly.

And by the term "belly fat" I don't just mean that outer layer of skin that you can "pinch" between your fingers – the way you might do on your hips or thighs. The belly fat I am talking about lies deep within your abdomen in a structure known as the "omentum". Normally, this is a thin layer of fat meant to surround and cushion your internal organs. But what happens when the "omentum" begins to accumulate too many fat cells?

First, that fat presses against and eventually entwines into your internal organs, so nothing works quite the way it should. But more importantly, this fatty layer begins to produce an enormous amount of inflammatory compounds - much more so than fat found anywhere else in your body. And this is where the real link to fertility problems begins. Why?

First, inflammation of any kind will contribute to and even worsen two of the most significant fertility robbing conditions in young women: The menstrual related disorder known as endometriosis, and PCOS or poly cystic ovary syndrome a condition closely linked to type 2 diabetes and insulin resistance.

If fact you have been diagnosed with either endometriosis or PCOS the inflammation produced by belly fat can not only contribute to your symptoms, but also make it much more difficult to overcome the fertility challenges posed by these conditions.

But even if you don't have either of these health problems, inflammation related to high levels of belly fat can still harm your fertility affecting ovulation as well as the transport of the embryo through your fallopian tubes to your uterus. In some women inflammation can even disrupt embryo implantation, increasing the risk of miscarriage.

In your partner, these same inflammatory compounds not only contribute to insulin resistance and ultimately type2 diabetes, but together with excess estrogen also produced by fat cells, seriously disrupts production of testosterone – which in turn can slow down or even bring his sperm production to a halt.

While certainly, losing weight anywhere on your body can help reduce the impact of inflammation and even reduce the amount of inflammatory chemicals produced overall, losing belly fat is perhaps the most beneficial to your fertility. In fact, even losing just a few pounds in this area can yield dramatic results for you and your partner.

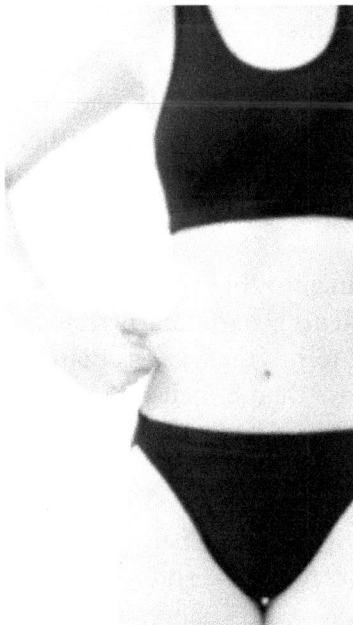

Take The Pinch Test!

If you can pinch more than inch of body fat, then you might have enough extra pounds to interfere with your fertility.

To do the Pinch Test: Locate the area just above your waist and literally "pinch" yourself. If what you feel extends out further than the first knuckle digit of your thumb, then you've pinched over an inch!

Remember however, loose skin doesn't count. In order to test body fat you have to actually feel a sense of thickness between your fingers.

Is Your Belly Just Plump – Or Dangerously Fat: How to Tell

Most women – particularly those who have given birth to a child in the past - have that all-too-familiar "pooch"-a little bit of a chubby belly that may even have a "jiggly" look and feel.

Men as well can put on a few pounds in the mid section and easily succumb to "muffin top" over their jeans!   While this may make it difficult to wear the latest fashions, generally speaking, neither of these scenarios represents true "belly fat" - but instead a little bit of outer fat mixed with some loose skin.

One way to know for certain, however, is to check your BMI or body mass index. This is a type of calculation that uses your weight and height to determine what the healthiest level of body fat should be. (See the BMI Calculator later in this chapter).

For most men and women of average height, a BMI over 30 suggests a serious weight problem – an issue that impacts over 30% of adults in the US today. Once your BMI creeps up to 40 and beyond, then overweight becomes "obese" – a term associated with a slew of health risks, including infertility.

But another way to tell if you or your partner are harboring the potentially dangerous "belly fat" is to simply look in the mirror and check your shapes.

If either of you see an "Apple" - a rounded shape through your middle, with little or no definition to your waist,   usually paired with thinner legs and arms - then it's highly likely you do have enough belly fat to interfere with your fertility, even if you are only a bit overweight.

If you are pear shaped - holding most of your weight in your thighs and rump – then you might also be holding significant belly fat as well. This is particularly true if your waist measurement is over 35 inches, or if your waist-to-hip ratio is less than 0.8. In fact, even if you are of normal weight, but there is less than 8 inches of difference between your hips and your waist then you may also be harboring some of this dangerous belly fat.

The good news: Not only will losing weight overall help to reduce belly fat, there are also a number of things you can do to specifically *target belly fat* – and a little later in this chapter you'll discover what really works!

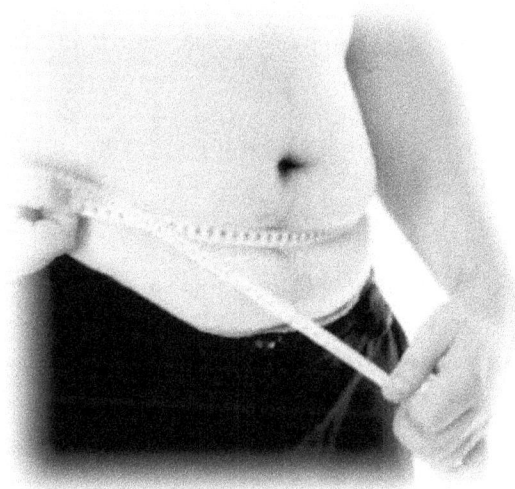

Hot Testicles, a Beer Belly and Male Infertility

Q: *We're trying to get pregnant and not having much luck. My husband has a bit of a "beer belly" and his doctor said it's responsible for his low sperm count – because his testicles are too hot. He said losing some weight could help us get pregnant. Can this be true?*

A: While I know it may sound strange, the truth is, that when a man carries a great deal of fat in his lower belly, he can literally be "smothering" his testicles every time he sits down! And this in turn can have a dramatic effect on sperm production. Why?

Sperm is heat sensitive – and when temperatures inside the testes rise too high, production slows down. If temperatures remain high for a long enough period of time, sperm production can stop completely.

Moreover, prolonged exposure to heat in the testicle region also impacts the epididymus – the part of the male reproductive system that helps sperm mature and learn to swim. When the epididymus becomes damaged it not only compromises a man's fertility but can also result in a higher percentage of deformed sperm .This, in turn, increases his partner's risk of miscarriage and his baby's risk of birth defects.

Although the most common causes of "hot testicles" are traditional heat sources – such as hot tubs, saunas, hot baths , electric blankets, or even laptop computers - certainly belly fat can contribute to this problem in a significant way.

While losing weight can help, your husband can help keep his sperm safe by simply wearing loose cool clothing whenever possible – particularly when exercising or doing any physical activity. The workout fabrics to avoid include tight, spandex shorts, synthetic fibers that don't breathe, tight fitting jeans with spandex (worn right after working out) or a tight spandex or nylon bikini .

What can also help: Avoiding tight underwear, and when at home, going without pants as much as possible. This will help to compensate for whatever heat buildup has occurred during the day.

While wearing boxer shorts instead of briefs can help making the switch a day or two before attempting conception won't make a difference since the sperm he is ejaculating today were actually made 11 to 12 weeks prior.

At the same time, however, if he is willing to begin making changes two to three months prior to when you want to get pregnant – including losing some of his "beer belly" and reducing heat exposure, it will definitely help maximize his sperm count when conception time rolls around.

Boxers Vs. Briefs

Q: *Any truth to the idea that men who wear boxer shorts are more fertile? Should I make my hubby switch?*

A: There's a reason this rumor has lasted longer than some medical discoveries! The truth is that because boxer shorts do allow more air to circulate in the genital area, at least theoretically they can keep the area cooler - and cooler testicles produce better sperm.

That said, a study published in the *Journal of Urology* recently found that men who wore briefs were not any more likely to have fertility problems than men who wore boxers.

Personally I have always believed that if you engage in activities that cause heat build-up in the testicle area (like bike riding or other vigorous sports) and particularly if you use a laptop computer *on your lap,* then wearing boxer shorts may be a good idea since it will allow whatever heat is generated to dissipate quicker - which means the testicles are exposed to heat for a shorter period of time. And that's good for fertility!

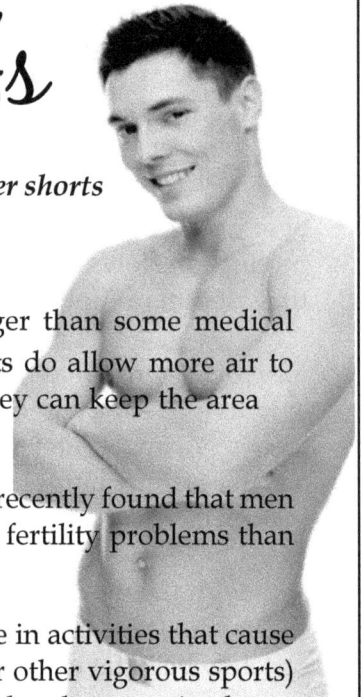

Your
Body Mass Index
Chart

Body Mass Index or BMI is way of using a person's height and weight to calculate their level of body fat. While a BMI calculation does not measure body fat directly, research shows the results correlate with those tests that do – such as underwater weighing, or a type of special x-ray known as absorptiometry (DXA).

Since however, both these tests can be expensive – and the BMI is free for anyone to use – it's easy to see why it's become one of the most popular forms of fat calculation.

Today, most doctors use a BMI measurement as a screening tool to help identify risks for certain weight-related diseases. As a fertility doctor I have also found the BMI helpful in identifying those women at risk for some specific weight - related fertility problems.

If you are actively trying to get pregnant, or if you're already having a problem conceiving, then you too can use your own personal BMI calculation to do the same.

The first step in the process is to find your BMI. While there is a mathematical formula you can use to calculate it out, I've gone ahead and done most of the work for you – and put the results in the table that follows.

To use it, all you need do is find your height (in inches) in the column to the left, then move your finger across the chart until you hit the weight (in pounds) that comes closest to what you weigh, rounding numbers up rather than down.

Once your finger hits that number, follow that column straight up to the top column labeled BMI. This will be your approximate BMI or body mass index.

Example: If your height is 64 " (5'4") and your weight is 143 pounds, your BMI would be approximately 25.

Once you know your BMI you can go on to the second chart, to discover your fertility risk evaluation.

BMI	19	20	21	22	23	24	25	26	27	28	29	30	35	40
Height	Weight(lbs.)													
4'10"	91	96	100	105	110	115	119	124	129	134	138	143	167	191
4'11"	94	99	104	109	114	119	124	128	133	138	143	148	173	198
5'0"	97	102	107	112	118	123	128	133	138	143	148	153	179	204
5'1"	100	106	111	116	122	127	132	137	143	148	153	158	185	211
5'2"	104	109	115	120	126	131	136	142	147	153	158	164	191	218
5'3"	107	113	118	124	130	135	141	146	152	158	163	169	197	225
5'4"	110	116	122	128	134	140	145	151	157	163	169	174	204	232
5'5"	114	120	126	132	138	144	150	156	162	168	174	180	210	240
5'6"	118	124	130	136	142	148	155	161	167	173	179	186	216	247
5'7"	121	127	134	140	146	153	159	166	172	178	185	191	223	255
5'8"	125	131	138	144	151	158	164	171	177	184	190	197	230	262
5'9"	128	135	142	149	155	162	169	176	182	189	196	203	236	270
5'10"	132	139	146	153	160	167	174	181	188	195	202	207	243	278
5'11"	136	143	150	157	165	172	179	186	193	200	208	215	250	286
6'0"	140	147	154	162	169	177	184	191	199	206	213	221	258	294
6'1"	144	151	159	166	174	182	189	197	204	212	219	227	265	302
6'2"	148	155	163	171	179	186	194	202	210	218	225	233	272	311
6'3"	152	160	168	176	184	192	200	208	216	224	232	240	279	319
6'4"	156	164	172	180	189	197	205	213	221	230	238	246	287	328

Using Your BMI to Determine Your Risk of Fertility Problems

Now that you know what your BMI is, it's time to use this information to access your weight- related fertility risks.   To help you do that, all BMI results fall in to one of 6 categories:

- Underweight
- Normal Weight
- Overweight
- Obese 1
- Obese 2
- Extremely Obese.

So the first step in determining your risks is to use the next chart to determine in which of these categories your BMI measurement falls. Because, however, it's not just your level of body fat that is important – but also where that fat is concentrated – the next step requires you to take one more measurement. Indeed, as you just read, body fat that is located in the belly region is particularly bad for your fertility, so I'm going to ask you grab a tape measure and determine whether your waist is greater than, equal to, or less than 35". (For men, by the way, that number increases to 40").

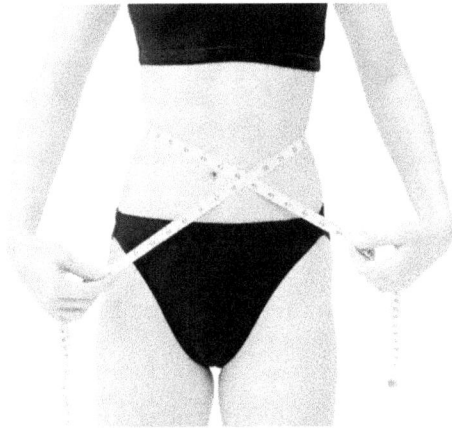

To Determine Your Weight Related Fertility Risk

Using the chart below, find your BMI in the column on the left, then follow across that line to determine your level of risk.

If your waist is 35" or less, stop at column number 3; if your waist is greater than 35", follow through to column 4.

Example: If your BMI is 26 and your waist is 33", your risk of a fertility problem is "increased". If your waist is 37" then your risk of fertility related problems is "high". Definition of probability odds:

Increased Risk: 50% or more likely to have a problem getting pregnant.
High Risk : 50 -75% likely to have a problem getting pregnant.
Very High Risk: 80% likely to have a problem getting pregnant.
Extremely High Risk: 90-100% likely to have a problem getting pregnant.

Risk of Weight-Related Fertility Problems

BMI	Weight Category	Waist less than or equal to 35 "	Waist greater than 35"
18.5 or less	Underweight	Increased	N/A
18.5 - 24.9	Normal	***	N/A
25.0 - 29.9	Overweight	Increased	High
30.0-34.9	Obese	High	Very High
35.9 - 39.9	Obese	Very High	Very High
40.0 or greater	Extremely Obese	Extremely high	Extremely high

Fitness & Fertility:
The Missing Link That Can Help You Get Pregnant

One important way to not just control your weight but also improve your fertility is, of course, to get enough exercise. Not only does physical activity help burn calories- which in turn often results in weight loss – it can also help you build muscles. Because muscle burns more calories – even when at rest – the more lean muscle mass your body has, the more calories you will continue to burn on an ongoing basis. And this normally results in better weight control.

But there is another reason why you and your partner should consider a regular fitness program: Working out can have a direct impact on both male and female fertility.

The reason? When you burn fat you also help reduce the estrogen overload in your body. Remember I told you how fat cells are like tiny chemical factories churning out a variety of compounds, including estrogen? Well, when you lose weight you autumatically reduce the number of chemical compounds fat cells are producing - including not only excess hormones like estrogen, but also other inflammatory chemicals linked to fertility.

But what if you or your partner are already thin and don't need to lose weight ? Research shows that even if you are at the correct weight,   regular exercise can still impact the production of inflammatory chemicals that are linked to fertility problems.

In one study published fairly recently in *the European Heart Journal,* a group of Finnish researchers found that the level of C-reactive protein or CRP (a marker for how much inflammation is present in your tissues and bloodstream) is much lower in people who exercise regularly. Moreover a group of Danish researchers found that exercise helps the body produce *anti-inflammatory* chemicals, compounds which are released by the bones and muscles while you are working out.

At the same time, other studies have suggested that participating in a regular fitness program can also help suppress the entire process necessary for creating inflammation – which is one reason why doctors now believe regular exercise is the key to preventing and even treating cardiovascular disease and type 2 diabetes.

So, if working out can reduce your body's ability to manufacture inflammatory compounds, and at the same time also create other compounds that help fight inflammation, it becomes a win-win situation not only for your good health, but also your fertility. This can be particularly true if you suffer from any inflammatory conditions that directly impact fertility such as endometriosis , PCOS or even insulin resistance or type 2 diabetes.

Your Metabolism and Your Fertility: An Important Connection

If you're already an avid exerciser - or even if you just take a run for the bus now and then - you already have some idea of how your body responds to physical activity: Your heart beats faster, blood rushes to your arms and legs, you probably feel a little warm and you may even begin to perspire. All these signs are indications that your body is working harder - with all systems running a little faster than usual.

But physical activity does more than just offer you a passing increase in physiological functions. It also has some lasting effects on what is called your "metabolism" - the rate at which your body processes everything from fat burning to energy consumption.

Command central for your metabolism is your thyroid gland, a tiny butterfly-shaped organ at the base of your neck. It is responsible for secreting a number of hormones which work in consort with your hypothalamus and pituitary glands to create a kind of "golden triangle" of hormonal activity that helps keep your metabolism working at the right speed.

When it does, calories are burned efficiently and more than enough energy is produced for all your body functions, including reproduction. But, all of this can change quite dramatically the minute your thyroid gland begins to malfunction. And here is where links to both exercise and fertility become apparent.

Indeed, whether due to illness, diet, or any other number of factors, when the function of your thyroid gland begins to either slow down or speed up , your entire body chemistry - including all hormonal activity linked to getting pregnant - can feel the consequences. What happens?

If your thyroid is overactive and your metabolism is running too high, you not only have difficulty maintaining a good fertility weight, more importantly your body simply does not utilize estrogen as efficiently as it should. This can sometimes result

---

Q: *How do I know I need a thyroid test?*

A: If you are having problems getting pregnant - particularly if you are overweight and tired all the time and you are also having a problem ovulating, it's important to talk to your doctor about a thyroid test.

---

in an insufficient uterine lining – meaning, if you do get pregnant you are at greater risk for miscarriage.

However, when it comes to *getting pregnant* it has been my experience that a far greater number of problems occur when your metabolism runs too slow – and your thyroid is under active. What happens when this occurs?

First, you will likely have some difficulty controlling your weight – which as you read earlier is a problem that comes with its own set of fertility consequences, including the production of inflammatory chemicals.

But perhaps more importantly, if your thyroid is working under par it sends a message to your brain that there is simply not enough energy in your body to support reproduction. Indeed, as levels of thyroid hormone decline it impacts the speed at which your body metabolizes all your sex hormones, including estrogen. This interferes with egg production and ovulation on several different levels.

At the same time, your hypothalamus and your pituitary glands (part of the "Golden Triangle" I mentioned earlier) sense the decline in your thyroid activity, and respond by trying to jump start your metabolism through the release of a hormone known as TRH or thyroid stimulating hormone.

Unfortunately, a surplus of TRH sends a message to your pituitary gland (also located in your brain) to release still one more chemical known as prolactin. This hormone suppresses the production of FSH and LH, which, as you read earlier are the compounds your ovaries need to begin egg production and eventually allow ovulation to occur.

When both FSH and LH are in short supply it becomes difficult or even impossible to produce or ovulate an egg – without which you cannot get pregnant.

How Exercise Can Help Boost Metabolism

As you read at the start of this section, regular physical activity can and does make a difference in how well your metabolism – and your thyroid gland – function. Indeed, research published in the journal *Neuroendocrinology Letters* in 2005 reports that not only does regular physical activity increase your metabolic rate, it also impacts the level of all hormones produced by your thyroid gland.

But perhaps even more important, exercise also helps to increase your body's *sensitivity* to thyroid hormone. And this in turn allows you to better utilize whatever amount of thyroid hormone you are producing naturally. This can be especially important if you are trying to lose weight in order to increase your fertility.

Indeed, when you restrict your caloric intake, your metabolism, and the entire functioning of your thyroid gland slows down to match it. While eating fewer calories can help you to lose some weight, because your body is now burning fewer calories, the loss won't be as great.

But by adding exercise into the equation, you can keep your metabolism going at a rate closer to how it worked when you were taking in more food . This means fat burning will be much more efficient – and you'll lose weight more easily.

Even more important exercise is a great way to *prevent* your metabolism from slowing down , and thus insure a healthy and normal flow of reproductive hormones – from brain chemicals like FSH and LH, to estrogen and progesterone.

The end result: When you do reach your ideal weight goal, your body will be primed and ready to get pregnant faster and easier.

Even better news: It doesn't take a lot of activity to keep your thyroid – and your fertility – humming along at the right speed. Studies show just 15 to 20 minutes per day is all you need!

The best exercises to improve thyroid function and help improve fertility:

Walking, swimming, running (in moderation) dancing, cycling or any type of circuit training. As long as the activity raises your heart rate by 30 to 50 beats per minute, then it's going to have an effect on your thyroid !

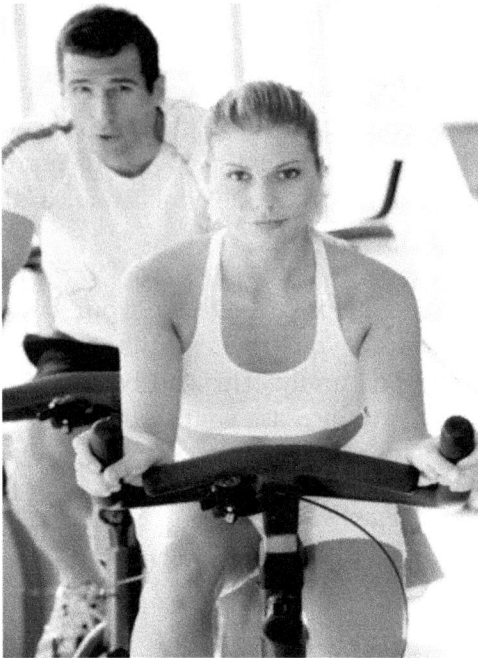

Writing Your Own Fertility Fitness Prescription: What Every Couple Needs To Know

When it comes to getting the most benefits out of exercise, studies show that moderation is the key. This is true when it comes to influencing all areas of your health but it is particularly true when you are trying to boost your fertility.

As you read earlier, working out too much – to the extent that professional dancers and athletes do, and sometimes, models who trying to control their weight – can do as much, or more damage to your fertility than not working out at all.

Of course I don't want you to take this as a "free pass " not to do any exercise! But at the same time, it's also important to remember that over-doing it has its own set of consequences, some of which can also impact your fertility. This is true whether you are working out too many days in a row, or if you are simply working out too hard and too long on the says you do exercise.

The general rule of thumb: If you come away from your workouts feeling exhausted and not refreshed, if you feel achy and sore and tired the next day, then you are doing too much, or what you are doing is too strenuous. While your body should feel some sense that you have worked out – perhaps a slight stiffness until you get going in the morning – you should not be in any significant pain either directly following your workout or the next day.

Another exercise golden rule: Give your body a chance to recover. The reason that most reputable coaches and trainers don't have their clients working out the same muscles every day is because your body does need time to recover . For most folks this translates into working out every other day three times a week.

If you do like to exercise and want to participate more often than that, then do what the trainers do and switch up your workouts so that different muscles are worked on different days. This will help prevent both soreness and injury and keep your body from responding to your workouts in a negative way.

Also remember that the same rules apply to both men and women. While men do have larger muscles and greater muscle mass in general – meaning their bodies can sometimes withstand greater stress - *still* the male reproductive system is far more fragile than many men realize. As such, doing the wrong exercises or working out too much can have some very detrimental effects on hormone production and even sperm production itself.

So, if your partner is going to the gym and working out every day – and he has been diagnosed with a low sperm count – then it may help to cut back on his workout time as well and develop a more moderate approach to fitness.

Working Out Together
Increases the Benefits

If you're used to working out alone - or your partner considers his 'gym time' as his only night out with the boys, then neither of you may have considered the benefits of working out together. And when it comes to your fertility, there could be a definite advantage in doing so! In fact, even though you and your partner may be at different competitive levels – and may not even enjoy the same types of workouts - it doesn't mean that you can't devote one of your 3 weekly sessions to working out together.

How exactly can this help? Among the most obvious is the continuation of the idea that runs throughout this book: The importance of working *together* towards becoming parents.

As I mentioned to you earlier in the book, too many times I have seen couples pull away from one another, and sometimes even attack each other when their pregnancy plans go temporarily awry.

For this reason I have made it a point to always encourage all my fertility patients to make getting pregnant a joint effort - one where you not only work together towards your goals – like, for example, eating a healthier diet – but that you also support each other in whatever individual goals each of you may have to accomplish.

More Excerise = Better Sex!

Studies show that men & women who exercise report having better and more frequent sex with their partners! When you do that exercise together, the benefits double!

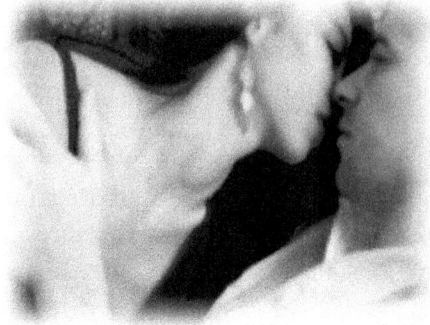

And when it comes to working out, doing it together offers a special kind of camaraderie that not only helps you to better achieve your goals, but in the process also grow closer to your partner – something that in the long and short run can have some great benefits on your fertility.

Moreover, in today's busy, crazy world filled with responsibilities for each of you, spending some time working out helps increase the amount of quality time you can spend together. In addition, it can also help you develop another common interest – an idea that studies show is of extreme importance when it comes to couple bonding.

Not only will sharing common interests and goals bring you closer together, but having those shared interests – and the time carved out to spend together each week – can also help you get over the occasional rough spots in your quest to get pregnant. Indeed, I have heard stories from many a couple who leave for the gym not speaking to one another – and return home arm –in-arm and ready for love, after spending this shared time together in physical activity.

One scientific reason behind this phenomenon is that exercise produces a series of brain chemicals that evoke feelings of happiness, relaxation and reduced stress – as well as increasing arousal and sex drive.

In fact, several studies have shown that men and women who exercise regularly report better (and more frequent) sex with their partners. When you're doing that exercise together, the effects can double!

Finally, each of you can be a source of support and encouragement for each other – particularly since nothing motivates us like praise from the one we love!

The Exercises That Boost Fertility: What To Do Together Or Alone

While it's true that certain types of exercises are definitely more beneficial than others what's most important is to do things that you enjoy.

So, if there is an exercise or a specific type of workout that you really love, then you should continue doing it – as long as you practice moderation.

Indeed, the fitness regimens that really work, are the ones you do. Remember, above all else, do what you enjoy and enjoy what you do!

That said, there are certain types of workouts that, for a number of reasons, appear to offer you not only a beneficial effect when it comes to getting pregnant, but also help you tone, condition and get your body ready for a healthy pregnancy.

These include exercises that are non-competitive, mildly aerobic (increasing your heart rate by 30 to 50 beats per minutes), and condition the entire body overall without taxing any one particular muscle group.

You also want to look for activities that you can do for an extended period of time (up to 40 minutes) without coming away feeling exhausted.

Among the best workouts that accomplish all these things - alone or with your partner – include:

- Swimming
- Power walking
- Dancing
- Cycling
- Moderate aerobics
- Stretching (which you should perform in conjunction with any workout).
- Tennis (in moderation only, in a non-competitive format)
- Multi activity circuit training (such as what is offered at Curves and many co-ed gyms)

To help ensure that whatever activity you chose always helps and never harms your fertility, I'd also like to take a moment to pass on these few simple guidelines – things that have always helped my patients make fitness a healthy and enjoyable part of their fertility plan!

- Whatever activity you choose, always practice moderation. When you are trying to get pregnant never exercise more than 3 days a week, and always make sure there is at least one day between workouts, necessary for your body to remain strong.

- Don't try to save time by doing all your exercises in one day. Instead, do multiple sessions on different days but keep each session under 40 minutes.

- Don't get compulsive – or competitive – with your fitness routines whether you are working out with your partner or a good friend. While one goal of working out is to build strong muscles and keep your body chemistry humming along, the other goal is to reduce stress. When you toss competition into the equation you defeat some of the purpose behind a stress reducing "fertility workout."

- Don't be afraid to cut back on – or even cut out - an activity that leaves you feeling drained and strained. While I don't advise you to suddenly stop all activity just because you want to get pregnant, I do encourage you to replace harder workouts with kinder, gentler workouts.

Finally, use the BMI chart from this chapter to monitor your weight loss and make sure exercise is not causing your fertility weight to drop too low.

If You or Your Partner Are Overweight ...

If you need to lose weight and want to use exercise to increase calorie burning, these same activities can work for you.

However, to turn them from fertility fitness workouts to fat burning activities, you need to do them a little more often and for slightly longer periods of time. If you can do more than one, and alternate them on different days, you may find you will achieve even greater fat burning potential.

What's important to remember, however, is that you don't want to work out to the point where you feel stressed and tired – because neither is good for fertility.

Moreover, if you or your partner are overweight and have not exercised for a while, then you need to start slow and build both your endurance and your muscle strength.

One of the best ways to do with is by walking. While power walking (a fast paced walk carrying up to two pound weights in each hand) adds some aerobic activity to the regimen that will burn more calories faster, it's also perfectly okay to stroll leisurely, focusing on building your stamina for distance. Indeed, studies show that just the simple activity of continuous walking for up to 20 minutes per day can reduce stress, help bring hormones into balance and improve circulation to vital organs, including your ovaries and uterus.

There is in fact significant research to show that when blood flow is increased to your reproductive organs, egg production and release occur on a timelier schedule.

If You Are Normal Weight or Underweight ...

If you or your partner are normal weight, or even weigh a bit less than average, your fertility can still benefit from regular moderate exercise!

In fact, I can't stress enough the importance of regular physical activity, no matter your shape or size.

Indeed, it has been my experience that many women who are underweight also suffer from a hormone imbalance that clearly affects fertility. And if this is the case for you – and particularly if your menstrual cycle is somewhat irregular - then certain fitness activities can work to help get your reproductive system back on track.

But even if you are of normal weight, with no health problems to interfere with fertility, regular exercise remains a key way for you and your partner to maintain your overall health – which is one of the best ways to insure your fertility.

If you don't need to lose weight, you should select activities that concentrate on muscle building and conditioning rather than fat burning.

This includes activities such as walking, weight training, stretching, Tai Chi, or particularly yoga. In fact, in the next chapter you will discover how yoga can be one of the universally best workouts for both male and female fertility – no matter your weight, shape or size.

Fertility , Weight and Fitness:
Some Final Words of Advice

There is no doubt in my mind that we are living in a culture where we tend to spend a lot more time sitting behind a desk (or as the case may be, on a couch propping up our laptop!) And while I wouldn't go so far as to say our inactivity as a nation is solely responsible for the increase in fertility problems, I do believe it plays an important role. When you combine a lack of activity with simply putting more food on our plate each day, it does become a recipe for a number of health problems - including infertility.

As such, I encourage each of you to not only eat healthy meals and enjoy a healthy lifestyle - but also to have an active life. While regular workouts scheduled on specific days at specific times is one way to ensure that this part of your life is not overlooked, it's not the only way to get activity into your life.

Indeed, walking the dog, going dancing on a Saturday night, taking your bike to the mall (instead of your car) or talking the stairs instead of the elevator very much count when it comes to enhancing your fertility.

 In fact, the more you move, the more you will enjoy moving – and this alone can help encourage a happy, positive state of mind. And that is guaranteed boost to your fertility.

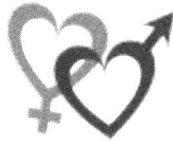

Chapter Seven

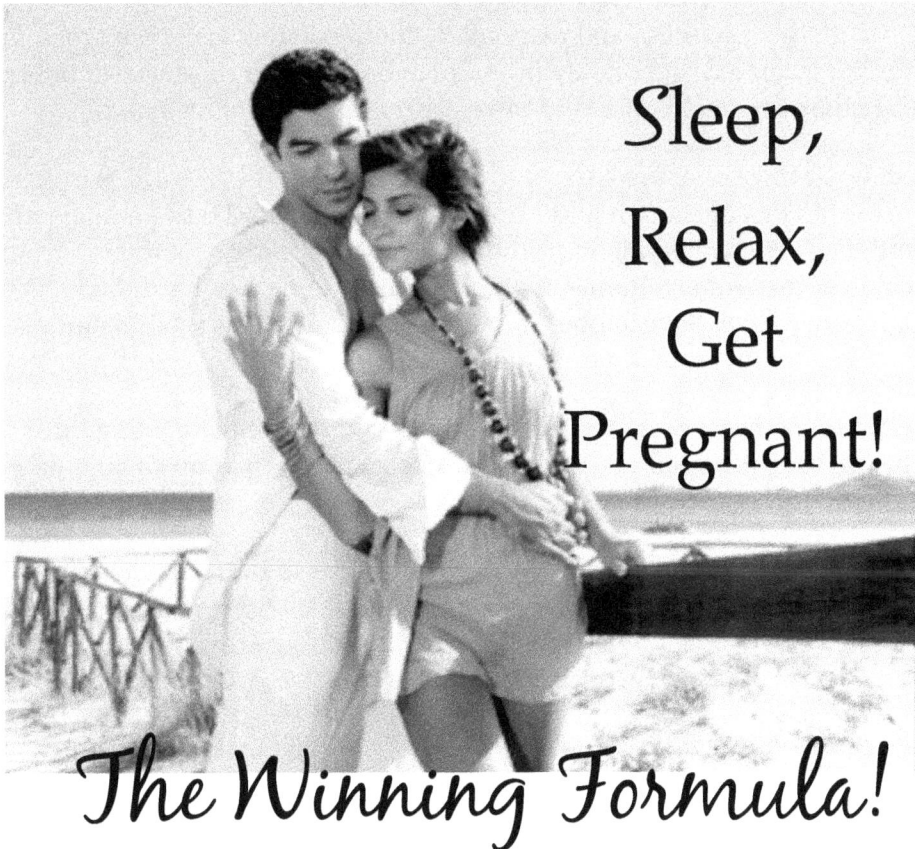

Sleep, Relax, Get Pregnant!

The Winning Formula!

If you've been trying to get pregnant for a while now – or even if you're still in the planning stages - you've no doubt heard at least one well meaning friend or family member tell you that the quickest way to get pregnant is to " let things happen naturally. "

Indeed, the idea of "trying too hard" has long been blamed when couples don't get pregnant as quickly as they thought they would. In fact, maybe even your own doctor has told you time and again to "Relax – stop worrying – and let nature take its course."

If you're like many of my patients, I'm sure you find this hard to believe! When we are living in an age where high tech medicine has taken getting pregnant to a whole new scientific level using something as simple as relaxation to help you conceive seems like it's out of another century!

But the truth is, relaxation – and particularly the alleviation of certain types of stress - can play a major role in not only preparing your body to *get pregnant*, but helping to ensure that your conception and your pregnancy are healthy as well.

Indeed, while most of us are so used to living in a stress-filled world, we often don't realize the toll that our rough-and-tumble lives take on our body – and in particular our fertility. From hampering egg production and stopping ovulation in women, to reducing sperm production and motility in men, to impacting the production of necessary reproductive hormones in both partners, acute as well as chronic stress can dampen fertility, sometimes to the point of infertility.

This is true whether you are trying to get pregnant naturally, or going through IVF or other fertility procedures. In fact, studies show that for up to 40% of couples diagnosed with "unexplained infertility", stress is a major contributing factor.

And when you think about it, it doesn't really seem so far-fetched. Over the past decade and particularly in the last five years we have discovered that many illnesses – including heart disease, high blood pressure, diabetes and even cancer – have roots in stress. In fact, today, 60% of all doctor visits are stress-related.

Moreover, when you realize that many of the same factors that link stress to these diseases are the same factors that can impact fertility, the connection becomes even more obvious and harder to ignore.

But what can be obvious under the scientific microscope can often be difficult to identify and deal with in real life. While you may acknowledge that stress *can* affect your health, realizing that *it's actually happening to you* is quite another story!

In fact, if you are like many of my patients, you and your partner may be so used to the feeling of being stressed out that the excesses in your life – and the stress that you are experiencing every day - seems *almost normal*. I believe that many of us have actually forgotten how it feels to be relaxed – and how our body responds when we are in that relaxed and calm state.

Moreover, if you have had some difficulty getting pregnant – or even if it's not happening as quickly as you would like, this too can add an extra layer of tension to your already stress-filled life.

According to California fertility therapist Ellen Golding, while most couples focus on the physical aspects of infertility, the mental health consequences are just as important.

"Infertility often makes women feel out of control – they become preoccupied with getting pregnant and that's all they can think of. It can be incredibly taxing, emotionally and mentally, on a woman's psyche," says Golding.

But getting back to a sense of "normalcy "– dealing with your feelings of stress about not getting pregnant while reducing the overall level of stress in your life can be key to a quicker and healthier conception. In one now-classic study conducted at Harvard University by Dr. Alice Domar, women who underwent stress reduction therapy while undergoing fertility treatments actually became pregnant quicker and easier than women who simply "suffered in silence" with the anxieties of trying to conceive.

This research led to other studies suggesting that any couple could increase their pregnancy rates when they took just a few small steps to counter the effects of stress in their lives. In fact, there is even research to show that reducing stress is an effective way to lower the risk of miscarriage and decrease the risk of premature births.

At the same time, I also know that simply telling you to slow down and relax is not going to do much to reduce your stress. In fact, for many couples, being told that stress can make it harder to get pregnant actually results in more stress – and an even harder time conceiving.

What really can help, however, is learning a bit more about how stress can impact fertility – and then using that knowledge to not only recognize the areas of your life that might be in line for some changes, but what you can do to make those changes come about.

Which is why as we continue our fertility journey, it's important that we take a few moments out to not just stop and smell the roses, but also understand how and why doing so can help us lead a healthier and more fertile life!

How Stress Affects Fertility: What You Should Know

Although research shows that there are a number of ways in which stress can impact fertility, among the most important – at least in terms of scientific study – involves the way natural bio-chemicals involved in the stress response actually impact the hormones necessary for conception.

It all goes something like this: When you are under chronic stress – or even low levels of stress for a prolonged period of time – you begin producing a hormone known as CRH – short for corticotropin releasing hormone.   Secreted by a tiny group of cells within the hypothalamus gland, (located in the center of your brain) CRH acts like a sort of biochemical messenger, sending a signal to your pituitary gland (located just below the hypothalamus)to release still another hormone – this one known as ACTH (adrenocorticotropic hormone).

A powerful peptide, ACTH travels quickly through your bloodstream until it reaches your adrenal glands - two small organs that sit just atop your kidneys. This, in turn, causes your adrenals to release still another hormone known as "cortisol". This is the classic "fight or flight" stress hormone that helps prepare the body to "do battle" with stressors.   And this is where the connection to fertility actually begins. How?

When your body remains flooded with these hormones – and your adrenal glands are continually being stimulated to produce cortisol – it sends a message to your brain that your body is engaged in battle and needs all necessary resources to fight.

In an effort to conserve all your resources and help your body do battle, your brain begins shutting down production of any hormones or peptides that aren't useful to combat the stressors. Among the network of compounds that receive the "turn off" message: FSH and LH, the hormones necessary for both egg and sperm production.

Certainly, on a short term basis, this "turn off" is actually a good thing – because it gives your body an extra boost of energy to overcome any immediate threat of harm.

Once the danger passes and your brain perceives that you are once again "safe", all hormonal activity returns to normal – including that involved in reproduction. While you may not be able to get pregnant quite so easily at the exact moment you or your partner are battling acute stress, once you calm down – and the stress goes away – all body functions return to normal, including reproduction.

This however changes – and quite dramatically – when your stress is chronic and ongoing. What happens then? Simply put, your body remains in a constant state of battle. And this means your brain never gets the "all clear" signal saying the danger has passed. The end result: It continues to put a damper on all "unnecessary" hormonal activity - and that includes the hormones necessary for getting pregnant.

"It is very adaptive to not be wasting resources on reproduction during times of acute stress, [so the body just] shuts down reproduction ….until the stress is gone," says Professor Daniela Kaufer, of the University of California at Berkeley, where she has studied the effects of stress on reproduction. "These functions", she says, "go back in evolution a very long time."

Indeed, as stress continues unabated in women, the hypothalamus gland suppresses production of a hormone known as GnRH – which as you read earlier in this book is necessary to kick off the production of both FSH and LH – the key hormones necessary for egg development, growth and release. In men, continued stress impacts the brain hormones which turn the production of testosterone on and off. And that means sperm production slows down – or can even stop.

In one medical review recently published in the *Australian and New Zealand Journal of Obstetrics and Gynaecology,* it was noted that men who are under stress are much more likely to suffer with poor semen quality. While severe depression has long been associated with reduced levels of testosterone, as this review points out, significant acute stress can have similar effects.

Moreover research has shown that both high levels of stress and anxiety can actually have a deteriorating effect on sperm, reducing sperm count, motility and even the percentage of healthy sperm that are produced. At least two studies have shown that when interventional steps are taken to decrease the anxiety, sperm parameters improve, and conception rates go up.

In addition, there isn't a man alive who hasn't experienced "performance anxiety" – a type of stress that affects his ability to have an erection. Today studies show that it's not just a bout of "performance anxiety" that can affect men in this way, but, when it goes on long enough, so can every day stress. So, even if your partner is producing sperm, high stress levels may keep him from being able to transport that sperm out of his body with enough force to send it traveling through your reproductive system so fertilization can take place.

Stress and the Anti-Fertility Hormone

Although the biochemistry produced by the stress response can, in and of itself, be harmful to fertility, there is still yet one more piece to this disturbing puzzle. In studies conducted by Professor Kaufer and published by the *National Academy of Sciences* we learned that when we are under stress our brain not only suppresses key reproductive hormones, it also begins boosting production of a tiny protein known as GnIH – or gonadatropin – inhibitory hormone – a natural biochemical that can be the real fertility enemy. Why?

GnIH not only suppresses production of GnRH (necessary to kick-start the production of FSH and LH) it also works to directly *lower production* of *all sex hormones* – including estrogen in women and testosterone in men.

When combined with the already devastating effects of stress hormones such as cortisol, the production of GnIH puts a kind of 'double whammy' on your fertility – one that can leave you and your partner unable to conceive without there being any identifiable physical cause.

Indeed, as I mentioned to you at the start of this chapter, for the overwhelming majority of couples who seek the help of a fertility specialist, no physical cause for

Women, Work, & Infertility

While both men and women are equally susceptible to work-related stresses, studies show that it is women who most often suffer fertility-related consequences as a result of a heavy workload.

In a new medical review published in the *Australian and New Zealand Journal of Obstetrics and Gynaecology* the authors pointed to a number of studies indicating lower pregnancy rates, lower live birth rates, and higher rates of miscarriage are associated with women who carry heavy workloads, particularly in stressful situations, or complicated by specific job stresses.

If you do have an extremely stressful job – and you can't do anything to change that – then it becomes even more important for you to reduce stress in other areas of your life that you can control. And a little later in this chapter you'll discover how to accomplish this.

their conception problems can be found. In fact, the most common diagnosis made by fertility experts today is that of "unexplained infertility". When this is the case, I and many others believe that this "unexplainable" factor can be easily identified and explained when you take a closer look at the stress factors involved in these couples lives.

The Stress of Getting Pregnant: What a New Study Reveals

Increasingly, many fertility experts have suspected that, over time, the struggle to get pregnant can create a unique stress of its own – making conception even harder. Most recently, we have begun to establish scientific proof that this is so.

In a new study published by a group of Oxford researchers in the prestigious journal *Fertility and Sterility* doctors proved that an enzyme which helps mark levels of stress was significantly higher in women who were having problems getting pregnant. That "marker" is an enzyme known as alpha amylase – and it's actually

Stress & Miscarriage

Although failure to get pregnant is one complication of stress, many studies now also suggest stress can increase the risk of miscarriage. This risk rises when stress hormones reduce the level of certain key proteins within the lining of your uterus – compounds that are critical to helping your uterus prepare a lining that is thick and healthy enough for a successful implantation.   When this doesn't occur, it can be very difficult for your fertilized egg to make a "home" in your womb.

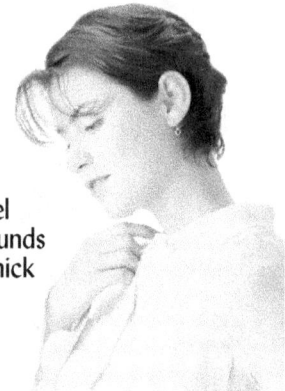

This is true whether you are trying to conceive naturally, or your eggs are being placed inside your uterus during an IVF procedure. Indeed, when the attachment to your body is weak and frail, your risk of miscarriage rises. I have also personally seen instances where stress causes a restriction of blood flow throughout the body – including the reproductive organs. When the uterus is continually deprived of adequate blood flow the risk of miscarriage also increases. Further, mothers who are chronically stressed both before and during their pregnancy are much more likely to go into premature labor and deliver a premature baby.

a natural body chemical we all have. However, when stress levels increase, we produce a chemical known as catecholamine, which in turn causes our level of alpha amylase to rise. As a recent study shows, together they form a very revealing "snapshot" of just how stressed our body is.

Indeed, in a recently conducted 6 month study doctors followed 274 couples all trying to get pregnant. None of the couples had any history of infertility problems, and all were told to use an at-home fertility kit to track their ovulation.   On the 6th day of each cycle the women also provided a saliva sample, which is the quickest and easiest way to measure levels of alpha-amylase, as well as the stress hormone cortisol.

What the study found: During any given menstrual cycle, the women with the highest levels of alpha-amylase were as much as 12% less likely to conceive, than women with the lowest levels.

While the researchers say they aren't quite sure how the enzyme correlates with conception problems, early evidence suggests that catecholamine –which also rises in response to stress – may reduce blood flow to the fallopian tubes, which in turn slows down the passage of a fertilized egg to the uterus. So by the time the embryo reaches the womb for implantation, it is simply "too old" to thrive.

As you just read, other theories suggest that high levels of stress hormones interfere with brain chemicals involved in orchestrating egg production and release - so when amylase markers are high it means other stress hormones are also in peak production. And this, in turn, can make egg production and ovulation less likely to occur.

Hidden Stress: Recognizing The Signs

Everyone experiences some stress every once in a while – this is a part of living! A bad day at the office, a fight with your in-laws, even a minor car accident can produce those quick, tumultuous bursts of stress that send your body reeling.

And while this can include an immediate effect on the production of fertility-related hormones, for the most part any negative effects resulting from acute stress, usually disappear within 24 to 48 hours, with no lasting impact.

This, however, is not the case when your stress is chronic or ongoing, or you continue to experience individual stressful experiences in rapid succession. In the UC Berkeley studies on the effects of stress on the hypothalamus gland doctors learned that the effects of fertility-inhibiting hormones can linger a lot longer when your stress hangs on. Not only do levels of stress hormones rise very high when your tension is chronic, the after-effects are widespread and lingering, impacting the entire cascade of hormonal activity necessary for reproduction.

This includes the production of GnIH – which as you read earlier is the "anti-fertility" hormone that makes getting pregnant extremely difficult.

So, the longer your stress goes on, the more likely it is that your reproductive hormones will be affected and the longer it will take for levels to return to normal.

What is most important about all of this is just how many of us are living with high levels of chronic stress and don't even realize it. Indeed, sometimes our lives can be filled with *so much* chronic tension that feeling stressed begins to feel "normal". In a sense, our mind and our body actually forgets what it feels like to *be* relaxed.

Moreover, whatever stresses that are present in our lives, they are no doubt made worse by the immediacy of the "do -it - now" society that has come of age in the 21st century. For example, while smart phones, netbooks and tablets, and the advent of social media such as Facebook, My Space, and Linked In have made our personal and business communications easier, they have also created the pressure *to communicate* – and to do so with astounding immediacy, to our friends, our family, even our boss or work colleagues.

For many of us the benefits that come with all these "smart" devices can be overshadowed by the stresses they can create. When we are unable to "turn off" the day at the end of the day, we also carry over many of our stresses, often without realizing we are doing so.

The worst part about this is, if you don't recognize your stress, you can't take the steps to reduce it! And since the effects of these hormones are cumulative – even when produced on a low but constant level - the longer your stress goes unrecognized and unresolved, the greater the impact on your fertility. Indeed, as you read earlier, one of the leading causes of "unexplained infertility" is, in fact, stress – or at least the hormonal upsets that occur when stress plays a continued role in our lives.

Combating Your Silent – *And Not So Silent* – Stresses

Whether or not you recognize the stress in your life, taking a little time out to relax – and taking some proactive steps to reduce stress levels overall – can have a positive effect, not just on your fertility but also on your general health.

In fact, I know many couples who, after engaging in just a few weeks of de-stressing activities saw a remarkable difference in their lives – not just in their physical health, but also their mental health. Many told me how much better and easier it was to relate to their partner when stress levels went down, and a great many commented on how much better their sex life had become, all thanks to reducing some of the stressors in their life.

The effects were particularly profound on those who weren't even aware that they had become so stressed!

Of course while reducing stress is an important component of enhancing your fertility and getting pregnant, I don't expect you to toss the smart phone, ditch the laptop, resign from Facebook and live in a grass hut for 6 months! Indeed, our way of life is *our way of life* – and there's not a lot we can really do to change that, and still remained connected in our universally connected world.

At the same time however, there are important ways to not just work around some of the stressors in your life, but actually incorporate specific "fertility anti-stressors" – into your everyday living. These are specific activities that have been not only shown to reduce stress, but also have some specific effects on fertility.

Certainly, as you read in an earlier chapter, exercise is one great way to reduce stress in your life. Studies show that working out just 20 to 30 minutes per day, 3 to 4 days per week can have a dramatic impact on the production of stress hormones – helping to keep levels low even in the face of continued tension.

But in addition to regular workouts, research shows where are also a number of other ways to combat stress and bring down the levels of harmful hormones that can interfere with fertility. As we go forward in this chapter I'm going to introduce you to some of these stress reducing methods and show you how easy it can be to incorporate them into your life - and in doing so help dramatically increase your chances for a healthy and fast conception.

Sleep, Stress & Getting Pregnant

There is, perhaps, nothing more relaxing than a long nap on a lazy Sunday afternoon. Toss in some sunshine, a hammock and maybe the sound of a light breeze whistling through the summer leaves and you can almost feel the tension melt away.

But it's not just the relaxing atmosphere that helps your stress dissolve. Study after study has shown that sleep is among the most relaxing and healing things you can do for your body!

In fact I am always amazed at how embarrassed and even ashamed some patients are to admit how relaxing a nap can be. When I would ask them what they do for relaxation, talking about activities like reading, gardening, exercising or even shopping seemed to come easy, while the idea of "napping" was somehow hard to admit.

And yet, the power of napping – along with the power of healthy, restful sleep – is one of the best things you can do for your health and for your fertility – not to mention your tension!

But how does sleep work its magic? And just how can it help you get pregnant?

Sleep more …
get pregnant
faster!

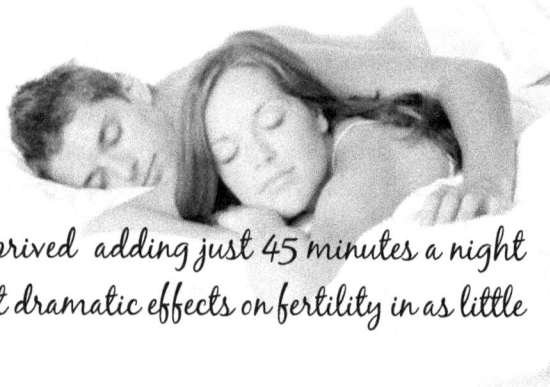

Studies show that if are sleep deprived adding just 45 minutes a night to your "sack time" can bring about dramatic effects on fertility in as little as one month!

In women, ovulation can become more normal; in men, sperm count can increase and there is often a higher percentage of healthy sperm available for conception.

First, when we sleep, we do more than just close our eyes and rest. Indeed, the entire process of sleep is one of restoration – a time when our body can wind down, our muscles can relax, our mind can turn off to the day's fears and worries.

But it's not just the relaxation of sleep that's important. Indeed, while we sleep an entire cascade of restorative hormonal activity occurs, at least some of which can counter the effects of stress we experience during our waking hours.

But the impact of sleep on fertility is even more direct than just helping to reduce stress. And it all revolves around a protein hormone known as "leptin".

As you read in the previous chapter on weight control, leptin is produced in our fat cells – and for the most part its job is to work in balance with another hormone known as "ghrelin" to help balance and control our appetite.

But leptin also has another job. Once it makes its way into the blood stream it heads straight for your hypothalamus gland, where it works as a kind of "light switch", turning on a whole cascade of hormonal functions, at least some of which are involved in fertility.

More importantly however, when leptin levels fall too low – which they can if you are underweight or overweight – at least some of those "switches" don't get turned on. And that means your fertility can suffer.

But it's not just weight that can impact leptin levels – so can sleep! Studies show that when you are sleep deprived, leptin levels fall dramatically. The longer you go without adequate sleep, the lower the levels can fall – sometimes to the point were almost no leptin is being produced at all.

If you want some immediate evidence of the link between leptin and sleep, think back to the last time you didn't get enough rest – and the morning and day that followed. If you're like most folks, it's a sure bet you were hungrier than normal the entire day, and probably had a stronger craving for sweets. That was leptin deprivation at work!

Moreover, the longer you go without adequate rest, the more likely you are to see your periods become irregular – and sometimes even stop altogether.

Indeed, many college girls who lose lots of sleep trying to balance the stresses of school work, a job, and social pressures often find their menstrual cycle can change dramatically or sometimes even stop completely, particularly around exam time, when sleep can be almost nonexistent.

And if all this were not enough, studies show that sleep – or more specifically a lack of it – impacts the production of a whole series of hormones directly linked to reproduction – including progesterone, estrogen, luteinizing hormone (LH) and follicle-stimulating hormone (FSH).

In fact, insomnia itself also has some impact on getting pregnant – and the key here is the stress hormone cortisol. As you read earlier, cortisol can have some damaging effects on a number of reproductive functions.

What happens when you don't get enough rest? Your body begins to literally pour out cortisol, all day long – which is one reason why you may be short-tempered and cranky when you don't get enough rest. That's the extra cortisol at work.

Adding to the impact: When we are sleep- deprived even small stresses can evoke a big reaction, causing still more cortisol to be produced. So, the less we sleep, the more stressed we become, and the harder it can be to get pregnant.

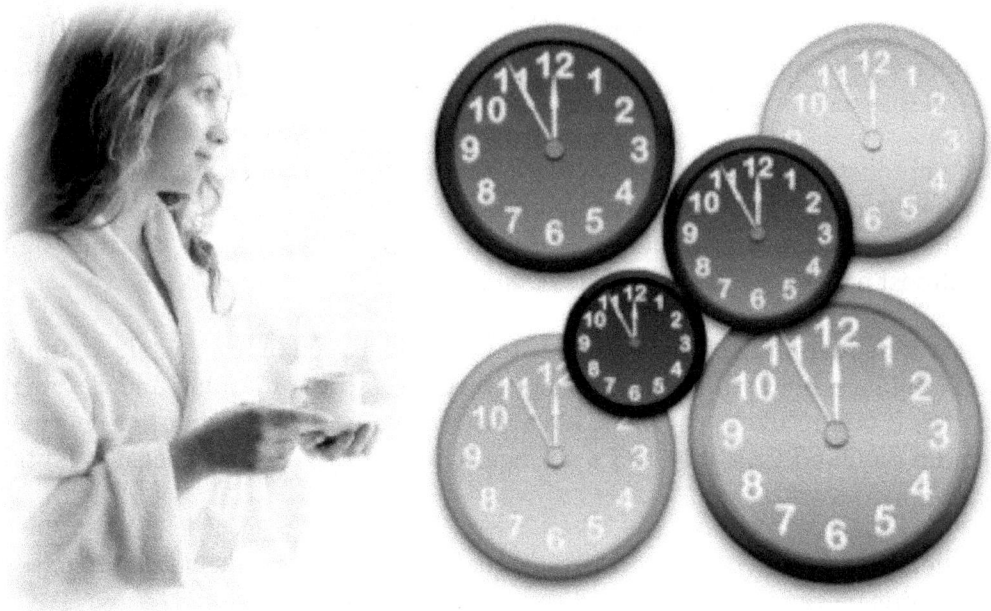

Working the "Infertility Shift":
How Night Work Affects Conception

When I was a young intern, just beginning my career in medicine, we had to work many long hours, and often times long overnight shifts of 16 hours or more. We used to call it the "graveyard" shift – a phrase which has its roots in the early 19th century.

It was during these early days of medicine that sometimes a person was incorrectly pronounced dead, when they really weren't. To ensure that no one was buried alive, each casket was equipped with a bell inside – and if the person woke they would ring the bell, thus calling attention to the fact that they were still alive. The cemetery caretakers who were put in charge of listening for those overnight bells were said to work the "grave yard shift".

Today, of course it simply means working a long over night shift, like we did as hospital interns. But it's not so much the long hours as it is the time frame that might affect fertility. Indeed, a number of studies have shown that night workers, particularly those assigned to shift work, (where working hours can change from day to day), are far more likely to suffer from fertility problems. And this is true for men as well as women.

The key to how and why we are affected has to do with something called the "circadian rhythm" – a natural "rhythm of life" that occurs in direct response to our exposure to light and darkness.

Through the production of a hormone known as "melatonin" – which is secreted in response to darkness and stops in response to light – our *circadian* rhythm helps establish a *natural body rhythm* that can impact how not only how well we cope with stress, but also influence how well our entire network of reproductive hormones functions.

In fact, studies show that the more chaotic and irregular your sleep-wake schedule, the more "out of sync" your circadian rhythms will be - which in turn can begin to impact natural hormone production body-wide. For many couples the end result of sleep deprivation is not just more feeling tired and stressed, but also difficulty in getting pregnant.

Sleep More – Get Pregnant Faster!

While your busy life and hectic lifestyle might make it hard to set aside 8 hours a night for sleep – and in fact you may be so used to going on just 5 or 6 hours you hardly notice it anymore – I can promise that increasing your sack time can have enormous benefits, on your health and your fertility. This is true even if your work shifts remain erratic.

In fact studies show that if you can increase your night's sleep by just 45 minutes over what you are getting now, and do so for just one month, you and your partner can see dramatic effects on your fertility. For you, ovulation can become more normal, and egg production more likely to occur during each and every cycle. For your partner, there is likely to be a higher percentage of healthy sperm with fewer defective sperm being made. For some men, studies show that getting more sleep might even bump up sperm count by a measurable level.

When combined, all these things mean a quicker and easier conception!

If you just can't manage to log in more zzz's at night, then let me enlighten you on the power of a nap! More and more research is showing that napping – even for just 15 minutes – can have amazing restorative powers on body and mind! In fact, much the way we have learned that exercise can be effective when practiced in small but regular "doses", we now know that sleep can work much the same way.

Indeed, at the most primitive level napping helps to reset the body's alert system – helping to reprogram some of the effects of sleep deprivation. While napping won't substitute for a good night's rest, studies show it can help improve memory and concentration, reduce stress, and even give a boost to the immune system – all of which can have important effects on fertility.

My Fertility Sleep Prescription: To help optimize your fertility – as well as maximize your good health – I recommend 7 to 8 hours of sleep a night, at least 5 nights a week. In fact, I would go so far as to say that if you are already dealing with an irregular menstrual cycle or infrequent ovulation, or if your partner has been diagnosed with a low, or even low-normal sperm count, then stepping it up to 9 hours of sleep a night may be even more beneficial.

If you find it is simply impossible to get this much sleep at night, then I do recommend regular napping of 15 to 20 minutes when you can, and logging in longer naps - as much as two hours if you can swing it – on the weekends. If you and your partner can take that nap together, so much the better! A warm embrace, or perhaps taking turns at giving each other a massage can help you not only relax, but *relax together* – which can provide a bonding experience that I believe can have some subtle but important effects on your fertility as well.

Fertility Stress Relief: East Meets West

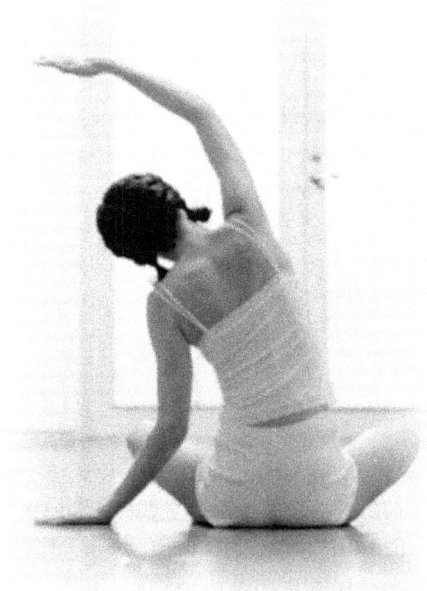

If I had to choose just one form of exercise that would universally help every woman trying to get pregnant, hands down, my choice would be yoga. Known as a type of "passive "exercise, yoga helps tone and condition the body via a series of postures (as opposed to movements) designed to strengthen and tone muscles.

But the latest studies show it can also have an enormous impact on fertility - related stress – so much so that women who practice yoga on a regular basis appear to be able to get pregnant faster and easier than those who don't.

Indeed, in the study on the biochemical side of stress that I mentioned earlier, the Oxford researchers suggest that among the best stress reduction strategies for countering the effects of fertility-robbing hormones are the ancient Chinese practices of yoga and meditation.

Indeed, the Oxford team found that yoga, alone or in conjunction with meditation, can actually change the body's chemical responses to stress. So, even if you are under tension, your body won't pour out the kind of harmful substances it normally does when stress levels rise.

Although Chinese Medicine doctors have, for centuries, been saying the same thing, we now have the western medical science to prove this is so. Indeed, a number of studies now suggest that yoga is one of the only forms of exercise to have beneficial effect on both fertility as well as pregnancy!

How Yoga Can Help You Get Pregnant

While most people think of yoga as a form of physical exercise - and some even regard it as a spiritual belief system - in reality it is a proven, scientific way of altering both brain and body chemistry.

Using a series of body positions, postures and "holds", yoga certainly helps tone the muscles, but in doing so it can have a remarkable effect on how we feel, not just physically, but also mentally. This, say experts is attributed to the idea that yoga can, moderate and even change the production of some brain chemicals involved in not just the stress response but also anxiety, mood, even depression.

When it comes to fertility, among the most important effects of regular yoga workouts is certainly the ability to reduce stress. But it's not just the feeling of being relaxed and more focused that can help you.

Indeed, studies show that the stress reduction achieved with yoga has a direct impact on your ability to get pregnant. The pathway is through the hypothalamus – the area of your brain from which all reproductive hormone activity originates.

As you have just learned, when stress levels are high your body produces a variety of chemicals and compounds that can dramatically interfere with the functioning of your hypothalamus, and in the process derail the brain and body chemistry necessary for reproduction.

Yoga: Good For
Male & Female Fertility!

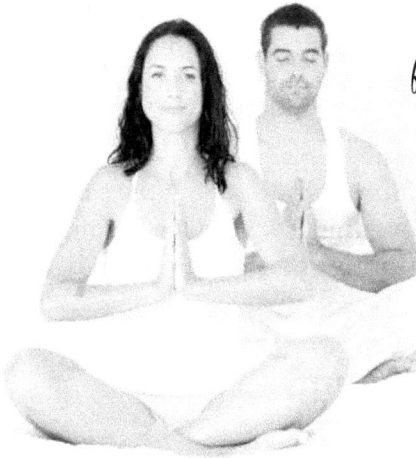

The same reasons that yoga can help female fertility - by reducing stress and increasing blood flow to reproduce organs, so too can it do the same for men!

Studies show that men who practice yoga have lower stress levels so testosterone production remains balanced. Practicing yoga on a regular basis can also help strengthen a weak libido and help certain types of erectile dysfunction.

Yoga works to not only to reduce levels of the stress hormones that might otherwise harm your fertility, but in doing so helps all your reproductive hormones work better and more efficiently. How?

Yoga is one of the fastest and easiest ways to improve circulation, with some of the postures and positions having a direct impact on increasing blood flow directly to your pelvis and all of your reproductive organs.

As yoga works to stretch and relax both muscles and connective tissue – particularly in the hips, groin, and lower back – blood flow to the entire pelvic region naturally increases at the same time.

This not only gives more life-giving oxygen to every cell, but it also helps to rapidly remove toxins and other nasty chemicals from your body, including those caused by stress. This, in turn, can lead to more efficient functioning of every organ in your reproductive system – and that can help you get pregnant faster.

Moreover, the practice of yoga also puts a unique emphasis on breathing, helping you to "tune in" to the rhythm of your body. (And you'll find a little more on links between deep breathing fertility in just a few minutes). When combined with the stretching movements of yoga, studies show rhythmic breathing helps release tension, which in turn reduces levels of the anti-fertility stress hormone cortisol.

In fact, the principals behind yoga are believed to be so effective in improving pregnancy odds, that today many fertility centers are recommending yoga classes as a way of increasing the success of procedures such as in vitro fertilization.

While many women still require medical interventions to overcome physiologic barriers to pregnancy (such as blocked fallopian tubes or ovarian malfunctions), yoga acts in ways that helps the body to work more efficiently and to better "accept" the fertility treatments.

This in turn increases the chance for a healthy pregnancy – without having to undergo numerous, costly treatments.

For women who don't have medical fertility problems, yoga works doubly well to encourage a faster, easier natural conception.

Not All Forms of Yoga Are Alike

As helpful as yoga can be, there are a number of different forms of this exercise, and not all are beneficial to fertility. For example, Ashtanga Yoga, also known as "power yoga" requires fast paced movements and advanced breathing skills that some of you may find stressful and difficult to perform.

Likewise, Bikram Yoga, which is practiced in near sauna-like high temperatures also focuses on more complex postures and breathing techniques.

For many women not conditioned to this type of activity, a Bikram workout is not only stressful but the high heat conditions could have an immediate negative impact on fertility. If you happen to already be pregnant and not know it, exposure to these high temperatures could increase your risk of miscarriage.

For most women trying to get pregnant, the most helpful form of yoga is Hatha Yoga, which is also the most common type practiced in the US.

However, be aware that Hatha yoga is also a generic term used to describe the movement and posture segments of all yoga workouts, so not all Hatha yoga classes are alike – with some much more complex than others.

Pregnancy Yoga To Enhance Fertility

If you are unable to find a Fertility Yoga class in your area, you can also benefit from yoga classes for women already pregnant.

Known as "Pregnancy Yoga" the postures and breathing techniques have been shown in studies to be the same as those used to encourage fertility. Plus, once you do get pregnant - you'll already be "with the program"!

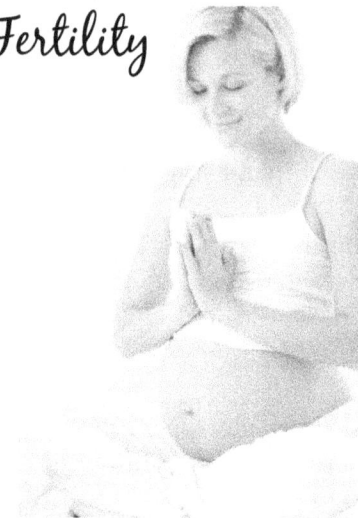

In fact, some Hatha yoga centers actually teach a fourth type of yoga known as "Iyengar". Depending on who is doing the teaching, this can be a mild and relaxing form of yoga or a bit more strenuous.

The best advice: If you want to use yoga to help you get pregnant faster, I suggest you look into one of the many programs now available around the country devoted to increasing your chances for pregnancy.

Known as " Fertility Yoga" or sometimes " Conception Yoga" or "Pregnancy Yoga", these programs are based on the postures and breathing techniques that medical studies have shown are the most likely to benefit women trying to conceive.

If you can't find a "Fertility Yoga" program in your area, then seek out a maternity yoga program – one designed to aid women who are already pregnant.

This will not only guarantee it will be a gentle program, but since many of the same postures and techniques that encourage a healthy pregnancy also encourage fertility, it can work to help you get pregnant.

Lastly, remember there are also find many books and DVDS featuring yoga for beginners and can teach you enough to put you on the right path to getting pregnant fast!

Prayer, Medication & Chanting:

The Antidotes To Modern Life?

As a fertility doctor and an obstetrician for decades, I can't begin to tell you how often I have heard phrases like "We are praying to get pregnant this month" or "We are praying for a healthy conception", or especially, "We are praying that we do not lose this baby."

Indeed, no matter your religion or your core beliefs, everyone, from time to time, experiences the strength that can come from sharing your burdens with a "higher power" - particularly when something so precious as the saving or the creation of human life is at stake.

But "praying" that everything works out okay is more than just a way of expressing your hopes and dreams. While there are no studies to show that prayer specifically increases fertility or makes getting pregnant any easier, there is quite a bit of research reporting that prayer can indeed have almost miraculous healing effects for some people.

In fact I vividly recall one couple who tried for many years to get pregnant and were unable to conceive. Just as they were about to give up hope, they went on a prayer trip to Jerusalem. Once there they became very devoted and prayed at length every day during their vacation. Upon their return to the US they visited me – and I was so happy to give them the good news: They were pregnant!

But apart from the miraculous aspects of prayer, when you look into the "science" you can see that it also has some medical effects . Prayer is, in fact, a form of meditation - a way of relaxing the body and the mind which in turn helps reduce the production of stress chemicals, including those that harm fertility.

Moreover, when we pray, we are acknowledging a higher power, and in doing so we unconsciously remove some of the burden of worry from our own shoulders. And that too can have remarkable, relaxing, stress reducing effects.

While prayer has been shown to help most in situations where there are already strong religious beliefs, there are studies to show that even those who are not dedicated believers can find some relief from anxiety and even depression through the power of prayer.

If you are suffering with fertility problems there are many religious-oriented organizations specifically for fertility support, some which also offer regular prayer groups.

While I don't want to give you the idea that you can "pray away" serious medical problems, I do want to impress upon you the power of prayer to help you cope, both physically and mentally with any of the stressors in your life –including the stress of trying to get pregnant.

Meditation and Chanting:
Two More Keys to Relaxation Success

Much like the power of prayer, meditation is a way to help quiet the mind, and in doing so also relieve some of the stresses of modern day living. Now if it sounds a bit too "new age" for you, I ask that you take just a moment to look at what the studies say – with an open mind! Indeed, published medical research has shown that meditating – which is really just the act of quieting the mind and focusing on nothing – can and does relieve stress.

And often, it can relieve the specific kind of stress that occurs when our mind is so focused on our fertility that without even realizing it, we are continuously worrying that a pregnancy won't occur. When this is the case, meditation can be one way to keep your *worries about getting pregnant* from actually stopping you from getting pregnant!

In one study conducted by fertility doctors in Barcelona Spain, researchers found that those who participated in relaxation therapies such as meditation prior to undergoing IVF, had a much higher rate of successful implantation, then those who didn't do anything to reduce their stress.

Writing in the *Journal of Human Reproduction* they suggest that in addition to improving quality of life, relaxation therapies – including both mediation and chanting – can have a direct impact on the rate of pregnancy.

In fact, many of my patients found that adding "Chanting" to their daily relaxation routines was also helpful. How does it work? Repetition is the key!

Studies show that almost any repetitive activity can help induce a state of relaxation that can actually change brain wave activity. Theoretically any repetitive activity can do it (its one reason why so many pregnant women take up knitting – the repetition is very relaxing). But when you combine repetition with the audible input of chanting, you get double the effect.

Indeed, research indicates that sounds produced while in a relaxed, meditative state can actually penetrate muscles, bones and organs causing cells to change in response to certain frequencies. Sound can also help stimulate the secretion of *stress-reducing* hormones and may even modify brain waves involved in the production of reproductive hormones.

So as long as you are chanting something positive, the overall effects should be good for your health and helpful to your fertility.

Mindful Meditation & Chanting for Fertility

If you've always wanted to try meditation but didn't know where or how to start, then a relatively simple method known "mindful mediation" might be right for you. To try this, sit in a comfortable chair and close your eyes. When you feel completely at ease, concentrate on the sound of your breathing. Breathe normally, but pay attention to each inhale and exhale. If your mind starts to wander (suddenly you find yourself thinking about that work project that's due or wondering if this is really going to help you get pregnant!) just keep bringing your concentration back to breathing.

If this seems too boring – and you find your mind being continually distracted – here is where chanting can help! By adding a word or a phrase to the rhythm of your breathing, and saying it, either out loud or to yourself as you breathe in and out, you can not only help break the boredom but also increase the effects of the meditation. For a doubly good effect, choose a short positive phrase that has to do with fertility – such as "Pregnancy Now" or "Happy Conception" or "Motherhood is coming". Say the phrase once while inhaling and once while exhaling – and try not to think about anything but the phrase and your breathing. Do this for up to 20 minutes once daily for optimum results.

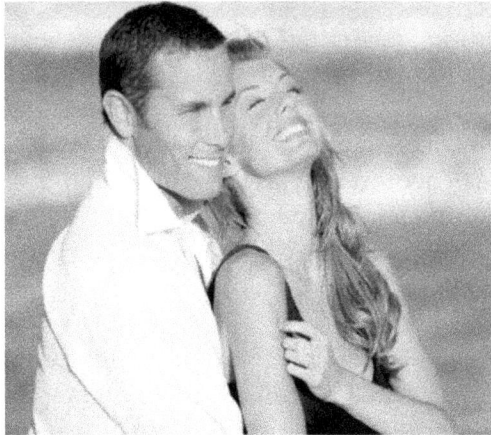

Reducing Stress in Your Life: Some Final Words

I can promise you that no one knows better than I how stressful life can be. This is true not only from the perspective of my own, hectic busy life, but even more so from what I see among my patients and friends. Life in the 21st century is, indeed, filled with stress – perhaps much more so than in any other century.

And all the gadgets and devices said to make our lives easier – like smart phones, netbooks, tablets and laptops? While it might make accomplishing some tasks quicker and easier, Web2.0 has also increased the demand for productivity that in many ways has added more stress to our lives. Just because you *can* do something faster, does not always mean you should!

At the same time I also realize that this has now become our way of life – and to ask you to change the world - or at least your world - just to get pregnant would not be fair – or right.

But what I do suggest is that now, more than ever, you consider the importance of making relaxation and stress reduction critical aspects of your health plan for better living . Doing so will not just affect your fertility but your every day health as well.

For this reason I urge you to do whatever you can to reduce some of the stresses in your life, particularly during the time frame in which you are trying to conceive. I know that doing so will make a positive and important difference in your ability to get pregnant, as well as help ensure a healthier pregnancy.

Certainly there are stresses – and stressful situations – which you are powerless to change. That impossible boss, nasty co-worker, meddling mother-in-law or maybe even an impossible landlord – all adding what can seem like immeasurable amounts of stress to your life. And I don't want you to feel more stress about not being able to change some of the things that, quite simply, are cast in stone!

At the same time, if you look into your life, I am quite certain that you will find many small stresses that can be either eliminated or reduced dramatically – and that, in turn, will allow your body more resources to cope with the bigger stresses you cannot change.

Moreover, when you combine this with anti-stress activities - things that can help reduce some of the physical ramifications of your stress - you will have a solid plan for reducing the tensions in your life, and moving forward with your conception plans in a much healthier and more productive way.

Remember, stress occurs in everyone's life. It's how we choose to deal with those stresses that make the real difference in how much – or how little – they will affect us. It is my hope that you and your partner will use the information in this book to make the right choices - those that will not only help you get pregnant, but also live a longer, healthier, happier life!

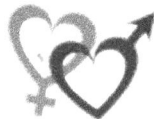

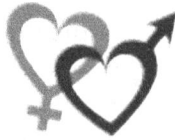

Chapter Eight

Every Day Ways
To Increase Fertility

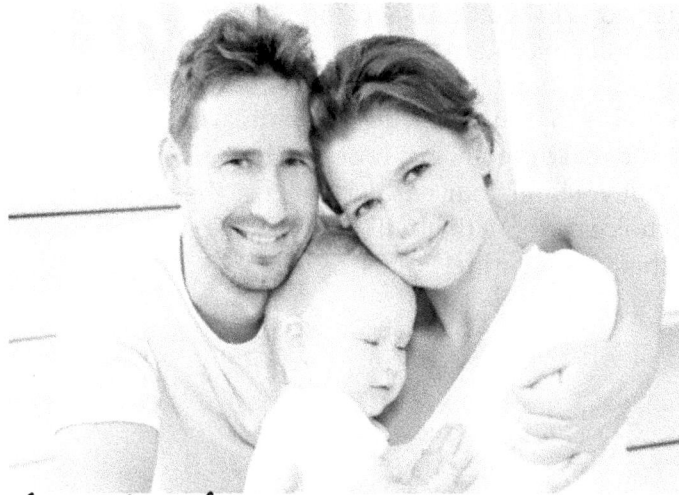

Lifestyle Choices & Getting Pregnant

Nothing is more natural, more beautiful or more wonderful than bringing a new life into the world. This is particularly true of a first pregnancy, but with each new child you conceive there is a unique and new sense of joy to experience.

And, if you are having problems getting pregnant - and particularly if you have been struggling for a while now - it's important that you never lose sight of the wonder and the joy of becoming parents – an opportunity I am certain lies just around the next "fertility bend".

Indeed by keeping your "eye on the prize", so to speak, you can continue to maintain the positive frame of mind which I believe is so vital to a successful conception. If you were to ever meet any of my patients they would tell you that my favorite phrase-and one in which I employ everyday in my own personal life - is "Never give up!"

But as important as it is to maintain a positive attitude, it's equally important to "back up" these positive thoughts with proactive steps to encourage, protect and enhance your fertility. Certainly, making the changes and modifications I have suggested in this book thus far – including those involving diet, nutrition and supplements – are among the most important proactive steps you can take.

Moreover, studies now show that there are, in fact, numerous aspects of your life and your lifestyle that, when, modified only slightly can also give an enormous boost to your fertility.

And in this chapter of *Eat, Love, Get Pregnant* this is exactly what you will discover – the everyday ways and the simple easy things you and your partner can do to increase your fertility and encourage a healthy conception.

Sounding the Smoke Alarm: Cigarettes and Fertility

I'm quite certain that you and your partner are aware of the many of the general health dangers linked to smoking. An increased risk of heart disease, high blood pressure and even cancer are all major diseases that can trace back to tobacco use.

But if you're like many of my patients you may be less familiar with the effects of smoking – and even the impact of second hand smoke – on fertility. And this is true not just for women, but also for men.

Indeed, in one study of nearly 15,000 women, doctors discovered that on average, those who smoke take up to 12 months longer to conceive than women who don't smoke What's more, the study found that problems are also dose-related: The more cigarettes a woman smokes the longer it can take her to get pregnant. For those of you who smoke a pack a day or more, the risk of not getting pregnant after 12 months of trying is a whopping 54% greater than it would be if you did not smoke.

But a delay in conception is not the only problem linked to smoking. For some women cigarettes can be a deciding factor in whether or not they get pregnant at all!

According to the American Society For Reproductive Medicine chemicals found in cigarette smoke are extremely toxic to a woman's ovaries, severely compromising her ability to get pregnant.

The good news: Quit smoking for just one month and your ovaries already begin the repair process necessary for a healthy conception!

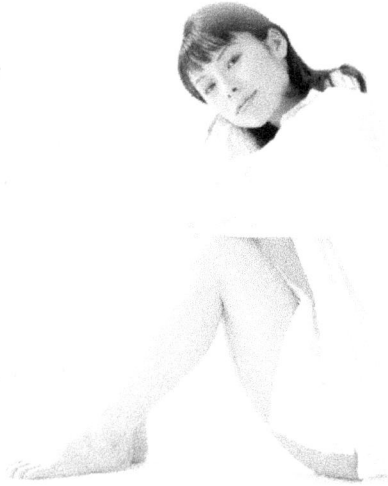

According to the American Society for Reproductive Medicine, chemicals found in cigarette smoke are extremely toxic to a woman's ovaries, working to kill off the tiny egg follicles or seeds inside that your body uses to manufacture eggs. The fewer eggs a woman can produce, the earlier she can begin to experience fertility problems.

Moreover, even if egg production does occur, toxic chemicals found in cigarette smoke could make that egg too unhealthy to survive fertilization. In at least one study on women smokers researchers found that the follicular fluid that naturally surrounds an egg was contaminated with the very same toxic chemicals found in cigarette smoke.

While smoking is bad for your health and bad for your fertility at any age, the risks take on even greater proportions once you hit age 35. Why? As you age, your follicle supply begins to naturally dwindle, so that your body is capable of making fewer and fewer eggs. Moreover, the eggs you do make are not quite as healthy as they were when you were young.

So, once you add smoking into this equation, you dramatically reduce your chances of conception even more. In fact, even if you are undergoing IVF treatments,

Quitting smoking before you get pregnant will not only help protect your health and your fertility, but also help ensure that the baby you conceive will be healthy and strong as well!

Studies show that the cleaner and more chemical-free a mother's body is prior to conception, the better the chance of giving birth to a strong, healthy baby!

So quit smoking now – for you and for your baby!

smoking still diminishes your chance for a successful pregnancy each time you try. Indeed, studies show smokers require *twice* the number of IVF cycles to get pregnant than non smokers, as well as requiring more fertility medications. Overall, women who smoke have lower levels of estrogen, fewer eggs available for fertilization and a higher rate of conception failure.

Moreover, if you do happen to get pregnant naturally, smoking also increases your risk of both ectopic (tubal) pregnancy and miscarriage, with the level of both chromosomal and DNA damage occurring in direct proportion to the number of cigarettes you smoke.

In fact, in the very latest study on this topic – the first ever comprehensive review of all major research published on smoking and pregnancy over the past 50 years – researchers found that unequivocally smoking during pregnancy is responsible for a range of serious birth defects including heart defects, missing/deformed limbs, clubfoot, gastrointestinal disorders, and facial disorders (including the eyes and a cleft lip/palate.)

The analysis, conducted by the March of Dimes and published in the journal *Human Reproduction* in July 2011, found smoking during pregnancy is also a risk factor for premature birth. Babies who survive the premature or low-birth-weight delivery are frequently plagued with other serious health problems throughout their life – including an increased risk of cerebral palsy, as well as learning disabilities and intellectual deficiencies. The analysis found smoking also increases the risk of infertility and stillbirth.

Since you could easily be pregnant 6, 8 or even 10 weeks before you know it, smoking while trying to get pregnant puts your health and your baby's life at risk.

Don't Let Your Partner's Fertility Go Up In Smoke!

Although female fertility is definitely compromised by smoking, it's not just women who are affected. Studies show the impact on male fertility may be even greater. In one analysis of 27 studies, researchers verified that men who smoke not only reduce their sperm count by as much as 25%, but that toxins in cigarette smoke also affect sperm motility. So, this means that the sperm which are produced don't swim as efficiently or as quickly – thus further reducing the chance for conception.

In fact, in one study conducted at the University of Buffalo, researchers found that men who were heavy tobacco users – which includes smoking both cigars and pipes and using chewing tobacco – experienced a significant drop in fertility overall . This say researcher is due mostly to the impact of the chemicals on sperms ability to stick to the outer shell of an egg - the first step necessary for fertilization to occur. Indeed, in men who smoke, sperm may reach the egg, but simply fall off once they get there.

Perhaps even more disturbing are the studies which show that if a smoker does conceive a child, the toxins found in cigarette smoke actually have the ability to penetrate each sperm and cause defects to the DNA – the "chromosomes" that form the basis of any child that is created.

While the degree of chromosomal damage in the sperm of smokers can vary widely, we do know that the more cigarettes a man smokes , the greater the chance that DNA damage will occur, and the greater the risk that this damaged DNA will be passed on to any baby he helps to create.

This can lead to any number of serious birth defects as well as an increase in several diseases that can occur later in the child's life.

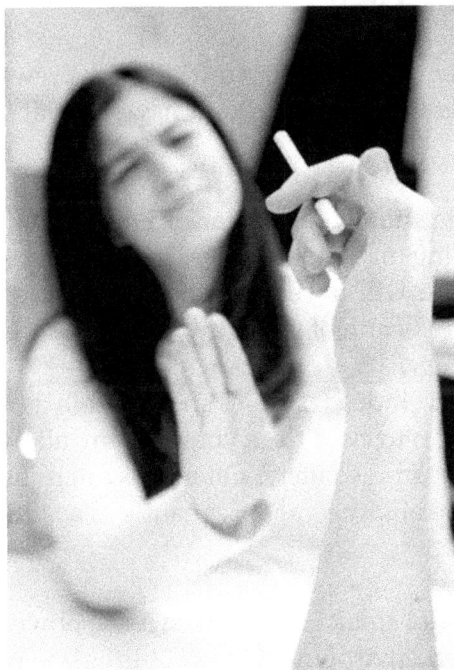

Q: *I don't smoke, but my husband does. He tries to smoke near an open window but I can still smell it - plus he also smokes in the car, which I also use.*

Can this kind of exposure to second-hand smoke cause me any fertility problems?

A: Studies show that even if you don't smoke, if you live or work in a smoke-filled environment, you can be affected as well.

Research suggests that women with partners who smoke experience the same delay in conception as women who smoke - so getting him to quit is not only important for his health and fertility but also vital for you as well.

While blowing the smoke out a window is helpful, if any of it comes back into the home the exposure can still cause you some harm – though it will be reduced since at least some of the toxins will be diluted when mixed with the outdoor air.

In the car, the effects may be more harmful particularly if you get in directly after he has smoked a cigarette. The chemical toxins can easily linger in the confined space of a car, as well as seep into car upholstery where they can continue to off-gas for a while.

A good barometer in either situation is your nose! If you can smell the smoke – either when he is puffing out the window or in the car – then there's a good chance that at least some residual toxins are getting to you.

The best advice: Try to get your husband to quit smoking. Not only is it affecting your health and your fertility, but he is also damaging his own. Once a baby is born, there should be no smoking in the home or in any vehicles where a child might be present. Damage to a child's lungs is immediate - and it takes *very little* exposure to cigarette smoke to cause serious harm to an infant.

The Good News: Smokers Can Turn Their Fertility Odds Around

As difficult as it can be to stop smoking, when it comes to your fertility the rewards of doing so are truly astounding. And the best part is, you don't have to wait very long to see the positive turn around!

In men, the impact of smoking on sperm will virtually disappear in 3 months or less after quitting. And because new sperm are being made every day, stopping smoking for even just a few weeks prior to conception will have overwhelmingly positive results - not only on his fertility, but the future health of the baby you will conceive.

In terms of *your* fertility, results are even faster! Indeed, studies show that in as little as 24 hours the toxins that impact fertility begin to clear from your system, allowing an important rebuilding process to begin almost immediately. Often, this can translate into increased fertility – and an increase in the ability to get pregnant – in as little as two weeks after you stop smoking!

The effects of reducing exposure to second hand smoke can be even more powerful. Indeed, removing yourself from a smoke-filled environment for as little as one week will have positive effects on your fertility. Stay away from second hand smoke for just a month and you dramatically increase your chances for a successful pregnancy!

Quitting Smoking: Some Tips and Advice

Certainly, quitting smoking is no easy feat. And for many of you it may take more than one attempt before you succeed. I f, i n fact, if you are having problems quitting, you should talk to your doctor about available treatments that could help you.

Although in the past, we often recommended certain nicotine replacement products such as the patch or gum, a new study has given us pause for concern about using these products during pregnancy, and while trying to conceive.

In research conducted at Loma Linda University School of Medicine and published in the *British Journal of Pharmacology* in July 2011, researchers suggested that nicotine in any form is harmful to a developing baby. More specifically when the mother ingests nicotine – be it from a cigarette or a nicotine replacement product – it causes the release of a chemical compound inside her developing baby's blood vessels. That compound changes the way the blood vessels react and in turn dramatically increases the child's risk for high blood pressure and heart disease – risks factors that are permanent and remain with the child for life.

Certainly, in the past we have recommended against nicotine nasal sprays and inhalants since both are categorized as Class D drugs and are considered unsafe to use during pregnancy. Because it's possible to be pregnant 6, 7 or even 8 weeks before you know it, it's also not a good idea to use these products while trying to conceive.

And while the new information on the nicotine gum and patches is still considered preliminary, I have always believed that when it comes to the health of an unborn child it's best to err on the side of caution. So I would recommend that you do not use any type of nicotine replacement product either while you are pregnant, or while trying to conceive – at least until we have more definitive evidence regarding the safety or dangers of these products.

So, what's the solution? I would suggest that you do everything you can to stop smoking *before* you start trying to conceive. In this way, you can safely use the nicotine replacement products without fear or worry. If you have already started trying to get pregnant, and are using these products right now, try reducing your intake as much as possible and if you can, stop using them.

You should also talk to your doctor about Zyban (bupropian), another smoking cessation product believed safe to use while trying to conceive. Although this same medication is also marketed as the antidepressant Wellbutrin, the form and dosage used for smoking cessation is somewhat different. As such it is categorized as a Class B drug making it relatively safe to use during pregnancy and safe to use while trying to conceive. That said it should only be used under a doctor's supervision.

The best news of all: If you have tried to quit smoking in the past and you have failed, your chances of doing so now are greater! Indeed, studies show that with each attempt to quit smoking, the chances of success increase.

What's also important to remember: Even cutting down the amount of cigarettes you smoke can have a positive impact on your fertility. Because so much of the damage is dose-related, the fewer cigarettes you and your partner smoke, the greater your chances of getting pregnant and having a healthy baby. So, while I strongly urge you to make "no smoking" your goal, as you head in that direction remember that cutting down can also help.

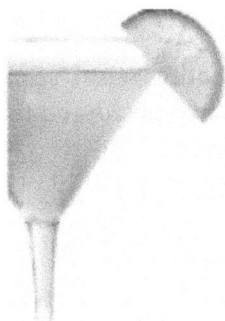

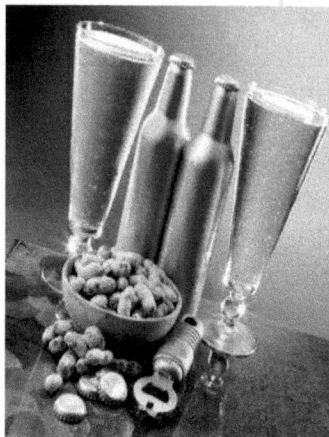

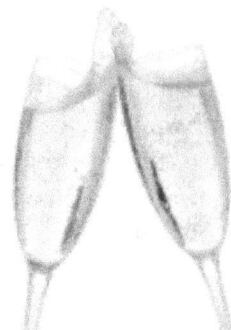

Martinis, Beer, Wine and Conception:
What You Need To Know

There's no question that over the past decade, and particularly in the past several years, links between alcohol and health have captured the headlines. From the heart-healthy powers of red wine, to the increase in B vitamins found in beer, to the blood vessel relaxing effects of almost any alcoholic drink, we now know that in moderation alcohol can have a powerful and healthy effect on the body.

When it comes to your fertility, however, the healthy links are not so clear cut. While some studies continue to report the health benefits of alcohol, others show it may be harmful. For example, a recent Swedish study of nearly 7,400 women revealed that as little as two drinks per day significantly decreased fertility when compared to women who had just one drink per day.

Conversely, a large self-reporting study of nearly 30,000 Danish women found that those who drank a glass of red wine a day got pregnant faster and easier than women who drank no alcohol!

Rounding out the confusion is an Italian study of nearly 1800 women who found no correlation of any kind between alcohol and fertility!

So, what's a gal to do? Certainly all alcohol intakes should be moderate - less than two drinks per day. But that said, since we do know that alcohol intake during pregnancy can be extremely harmful to your baby, again, I prefer to err on the side of caution and recommend against alcohol consumption while trying conceiving. Since it's possible to be pregnant weeks before you know it, abstaining from alcohol while trying to conceive is one way to give your baby the absolute best start in life possible!

If you find that eliminating alcohol completely is not an option, red wine is among your best choices, followed by white wine and champagne. If you can, avoid hard liquor.

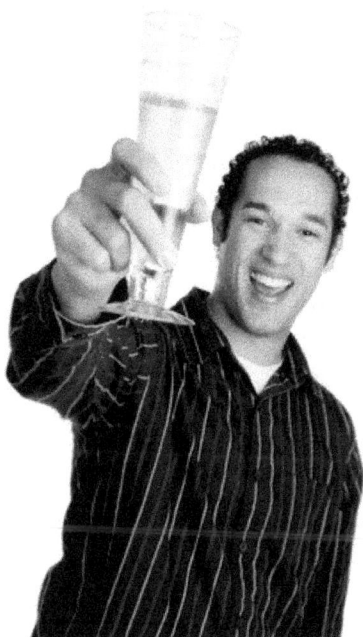

Alcohol and Male Fertility: What Your Partner Must Know

While the evidence linking alcohol and fertility problems in women is still considered preliminary, the same is not true for your partner. Indeed, the information we have on alcohol and male fertility is not only more concrete it's significantly more alarming - mostly because the effects can be so immediate.

Indeed, within 24 hours after becoming intoxicated studies show that sperm count can drop as much as 50%. In one study, conception was reduced by about 50% when attempted 24 hours after a male partner consumed enough alcohol to be considered "drunk".

But it's not just the short term and immediate effects that are of concern. When consumed on a regular basis, and particularly to excess, alcohol can affect the entire network of hormones necessary for healthy sperm production. This includes testosterone, the "male" hormone made inside the testicles and key to not only sperm production but also male sex drive. This is one reason why men who drink a lot often lose their desire for sex and/or their ability to have an erection.

Moreover, certain types of drinks may have an even greater impact on testosterone production, over and above their alcohol content. In several new studies conducted by the Medical Research Council in Cambridge, England, researchers found that both beer and red wine may be especially harmful to sperm – and that the harm can be further increased by adding a handful of the peanuts so frequently served at bars.

Indeed, researchers found that both red wine and brown ale, along with peanuts, were loaded with phytoestrogens – a form of plant estrogen that can reduce sperm count and in some instances, even cause estrogen levels to overtake testosterone levels. When this happens, sperm can no longer be effectively produced.

As such, if your partner can't give up alcohol completely, he should definitely try to avoid beer and red wine, as well as peanuts, while you are trying to conceive.

Reversing Alcohol's Effects:
It's Fast and Easier Than You Think!

What's important to remember is that as dramatic as the effects of alcohol can be on male fertility, reversing the damage is equally dramatic – because it can happen so quickly!

In fact, research indicates that avoiding alcohol for just 3 months can dramatically increase your partner's sperm count – to the point where some men can go from infertile to fertile! In fact, if your partner has been tested and his sperm count was found to be borderline low or even very low, I recommend that he abstain from all alcohol use for two to three months, and then have his sperm count checked again.

You may both be surprised to discover that his fertility problems have self-corrected. If, at the same time, your partner also improves his diet and stocks up on the fertility nutrients I mentioned to you earlier, he can not only halt most sperm–production problems, but sometimes even reverse some of the alcohol-induced damage done to his reproductive system. How can this help?

When the body metabolizes alcohol, the by-product is the production of cell-damaging molecules known as "oxidants. In men who are very heavy drinkers damage can extend to the tissues within the testicles, making it extremely difficult or even impossible to produce sperm in any significant quantity.

One way to combat problems is to make certain your partner eats lots of foods containing "antioxidants' – nutrients that protect fertility by fighting cell damage caused by oxidation. As you read earlier, foods high in antioxidants include most fruits and vegetables but particularly blueberries.

As I also pointed out earlier, your partner should consider taking a good multivitamin high in antioxidant nutrients such as vitamins A, C, D, and E. This can help prevent a condition known as "oxidative stress" – which in turn can also protect against cell damage that might otherwise harm his sperm.

Indeed, if your partner sticks to the healthy eating plan featured at the start of this book, he can not only build his defense against alcohol-related sperm damage, but also increase the health and the strength of his fertility overall.

Coffee, Soda, Tea and Fertility: How Caffeine Affects Conception

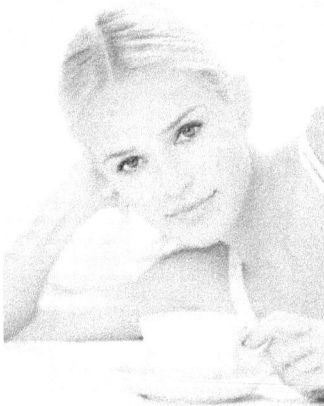

If you or your partner just can't think of starting the day without a steaming cup of coffee, and if either of you can't get through the day without at least a few energy jolts from either more coffee or other high-caffeine beverages and energy drinks, then you already know the power this natural stimulant can have.

And, in moderate amounts, caffeine is okay. In fact, in smaller doses it's actually good for your health! At the same time, if you consume too much caffeine not only do you lose the health benefits, but you can also create certain health *problems,* including some that impact fertility.

How do high levels of caffeine affect your ability to get pregnant? In women, problems occur due to caffeine's ability to dramatically increase circulating levels of estrogen.

Certainly, if you are estrogen deficient, this might not be a bad thing. However, if you have even a slight hormone imbalance (a very common occurrence in women of childbearing age) then caffeine just might throw your reproductive hormones into a tailspin.   When it does, your periods may become irregular, your ovulation can go off track, and ultimately you may   derail or at least delay your ability to get pregnant. Indeed one study published in the *Journal of Epidemiology* reported that women who drank 5 cups of coffee a day or more were more likely to have problems conceiving than women who drank less.

Moreover, if you suffer with even mild endometriosis (a menstrual related disorder and a major cause of infertility) I have found that the caffeine found in just one or two cups of coffee can worsen this condition and in doing so dramatically increase your risk of infertility.

Studies also show that high levels of caffeine can increase the risk of tubal factor infertility. While the exact cause isn't known, my hunch has always been that the stimulation of the caffeine causes spasms within the fallopian tubes that can push a newly fertilized egg to the womb too quickly – before conditions are right for implantation.

And indeed, some studies do show that high levels of caffeine intake early in pregnancy may increase the risk of miscarriage.

But it's not just *your fertility* that is at risk. A high intake of caffeine can also disrupt your partner's ability to make healthy sperm.

In one recent study on more than 2,500 Danish men, researchers found that those men who consumed more than 800 mg of caffeine daily - or about 14 one-liter bottles of cola a week - had lower sperm counts *and* lower overall sperm concentrations then men who consumed more moderate levels of caffeine.

The findings, published in the *American Journal of Epidemiology* did not suggest whether the caffeine in coffee or tea had the same effect. The researchers also pointed out that other components of the soft drinks – like high fructose corn syrup – could have also been a contributing factor to the impact on sperm.

Still, the effects of excess caffeine cannot be discounted as one cause of low sperm count.

Have Your Caffeine – and Keep Your Fertility Healthy

The key to keeping your favorite caffeine-rich beverages on the menu without harming your fertility clearly lies in the amount you consume each day. As I said earlier, a little bit of caffeine may actually offer you significant health benefits – so I don't suggest that you cut it out completely.

What I do recommend is that you and your partner moderate your intake, being certain to count all sources of caffeine. (And in just a minute I'm going to tell you about the hidden sources of caffeine in many foods and beverages).

So, *what is the amount of caffeine considered "safe" while trying to conceive?*

For Women: Keeping caffeine intake between 300 mg and 500 mg a day (equal to about 3 to 5 cups of coffee) will help ensure that your fertility is not affected. If you can stick to the limit recommended by the March of Dimes – which is the caffeine equal to 2 cups of coffee a day – you'll be doing even more to help encourage a quick and healthy pregnancy.

For Men: Up to 3 cups of coffee or per day or two 12 ounce cans of caffeinated soda per day should be safe to consume. However, if your sperm count is already low, I would recommend no more than 1 cup of coffee or one caffeinated soda daily.

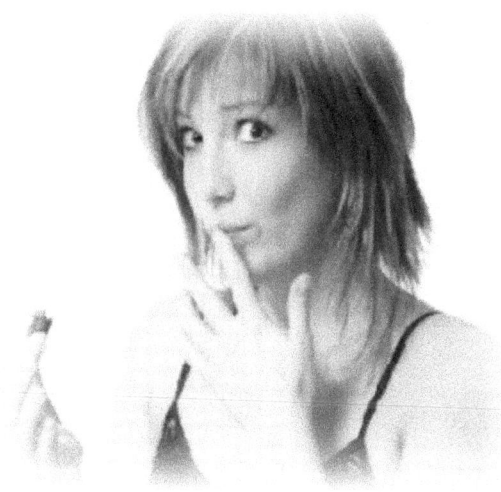

The Hidden Caffeine in Your Daily Life

While you may be limiting your intake of coffee, it's important to realize this may not the only source of caffeine in your diet.

In fact, most people do not realize how many unsuspecting foods, drinks or even medications contain this compound.

For example, many sports drinks and high energy drinks are loaded with caffeine, as are many sodas including Coke, Pepsi, and Mountain Dew.

Tea and chocolate both contain caffeine as do some over-the-counter headache remedies or menstrual pain products.

To help you gauge how much caffeine you are getting, I've put together the following list of foods and drinks.

Remember, your maximum daily target is no more than 500 mg total, and if you can stay below 300 mg you'll definitely give your fertility a boost!

The Caffeine In Your Daily Life

Coffee:

- Drip (8 oz) = 234 mg
- Percolated (8 oz) = 176 mg
- Regular instant (8 oz) = 85 mg
- Decaffeinated instant (8 oz) = 3 mg
- Expresso (1 -2 oz) = 45 to 100 mg
- Starbucks grande (16 oz) = 330 mg

Tea:

- 1 minute brew = 9 to 33 mg
- 3 minute brew = 20 to 46 mg
- Instant = 12 to 28 mg
- Canned ice tea (12 ounces) = 22 to 36 mg
- Snapple Flavored Teas (Reg. or Diet) 31.5
- Nestea Sweet Iced Tea -26.5
- Nestea Unsweetened Iced Tea - 26.0
- Lipton Diet Green Tea with Citrus (16.9 oz)23.0

Energy Drinks:

- Red Bull (8.2 oz) - 80.0
- Jolt - 71.2
- Mountain Dew Code Red – 55 mg
- Kick Citrus 54 mg
- Surge : 51 mg
- Mellow Yellow – 52.8 mg
- Red Flash- 40.0
- Big Red- 38 mg

Soft Drinks: (12 ounce serving)

- Pepsi One - 55.5
- Mountain Dew - 55.0
- Tab - 46.8
- Diet Coke - 45.6
- Shasta Cola - 44.4
- Shasta Diet Cola - 44.4
- RC Cola -- 43.0
- Diet RC - 43.0
- Dr. Pepper (diet and regular) - 41.0
- Diet Sunkist Orange - 41.0
- Sunkist Orange 40.0
- Pepsi-Cola - 37.5
- Diet Pepsi - 36.0
- Coca-Cola Zero - 35.0
- Coca-Cola Classic - 34.0
- Cherry , Lemon or Vanilla Coke - 34.0
- Canada Dry Cola 30.0
- A&W Creme Soda 29.0

Although foods like chocolate, tea or cola have far less caffeine than a cup of coffee, remember that every little bit counts and the effects on fertility can be cumulative.

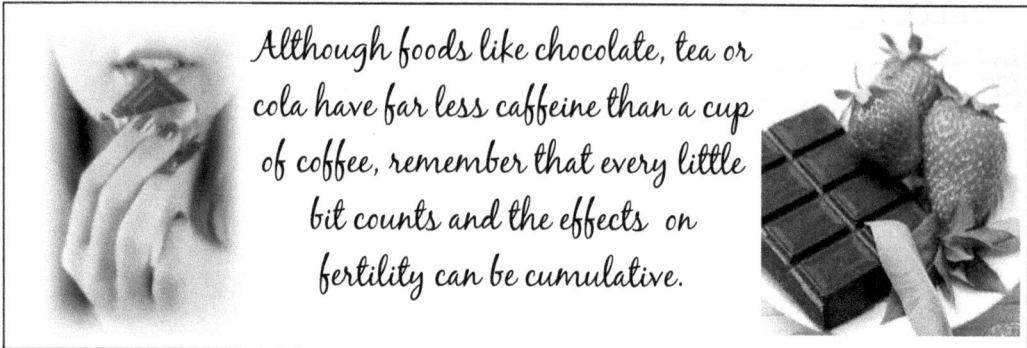

Cocoa and chocolate:

- Cocoa from mix (6 oz) = 10 mg
- Milk chocolate (1 oz) = 6 mg
- Baking chocolate (1 oz) = 35 mg

Over the Counter Medicines Containing Caffeine:

- Excedrin, extra strength,

- Maximum Strength Midol

- Vanquish

- Anacin

- Amaphen

- Dexatrim (diet pill)

- No Doz (wake up pill)

- Efed II (energy pill)

Also be aware that some herbal energy products contain as much as 200 mg of caffeine or more per dose, so do check the label to know for sure.

Your Medicine Chest:
The Prescription Drugs That Impact Fertility

I've always believed that it's important to approach conception with a body that is as free and clear of as many chemicals and toxins as is possible – advice that extends to both men and women. This includes not only the obvious exposures to harmful chemicals – like cigarette smoke, industrial pollutants and pesticides - but also the "chemicals" we come across in our everyday life – including those added to our foods.

But this "clear and clean" philosophy also applies to something else: The products in our medicine chest – some of which can have a downright nasty effect on fertility.

Certainly, there are some of you for whom prescription medications are a lifesaving necessity – and some for whom over-the-counter drugs such as allergy medications or pain relievers are needed to help you get through the day. And by no means am I suggesting that you forgo the use of *any* medications that are essential to your good health. In fact, when taken correctly, most medications in use today will not interfere with your ability to get pregnant – particularly if they are used on a short basis.

That said there are a few precautions concerning the way in which certain drugs can interfere with fertility. As such, it's always a good idea for both you and your partner to let your doctors know that you are trying to get pregnant, and ask if any of the medications you are taking could interfere with your fertility.

You can both also talk to your local pharmacist, who is an excellent source of information on drug side effects and interactions. If you have all your prescriptions filled in one place, then speak to your pharmacist confidentially and ask her or him to review your medication list to see if anything you are taking could interfere with your ability to get pregnant – and make sure your partner does the same as well. If you have prescriptions filled by more than one pharmacy, compile a list, along with a list of any over-the-counter drugs you or your partner use on a regular or semi-regular basis, and ask your doctor or trusted pharmacist to review it with an eye towards protecting and encouraging fertility.

To help get you started looking in the right direction, below are the major categories of medications known to impact female fertility, followed by a list of the medications known to impact male fertility. Remember, however, that every person's body is different, and much of the effects are dose-related. Also remember that not every drug in these categories can cause problems with fertility so it's important that you do not stop taking any medication prescribed or recommended by your doctor until you speak with him or her first. I can't emphasize this enough, particularly for those of you who may have a chronic health concern.

It's also important to note that if you are taking a prescription medicine, and it falls into one of the drug categories specified below, you should talk to your doctor to find out specifically if the medication you are taking could impact your fertility. If it does, then discuss what other medication with perhaps a lesser, or even no impact on fertility could be safely substituted.

You can also make use of the Internet, by Googling each of the drugs you are taking to see if they have any impact on fertility. If they do, then again, your doctor is your best resource in helping you find alternate medications that may have a lesser effect.

Drug Categories That Impact Female Fertility

- Antidepressants

- Pain Relievers (see below)

- Thyroid medication

- Antibiotics

- Gastrointestinal aids

- Older blood pressure medications

- Allergy pills

- Cold and cough remedies

- Steroid drugs (such as prednisone)

- Epilepsy Drugs (particularly carbamazepine and valproate).

Even if you or your partner believe a medication may be interfering with your fertility, always talk to your doctor before stopping any treatment.

Frequently there is another medication that can be safely substituted - but only your doctor will know for sure.

Drug Categories That Impact Male Fertility

- Blood pressure medications including Thiazide diuretics, spironolactone, aldactone, beta blockers, calcium channel blockers, alpha blockers.

- Mental Health Drugs – such as anti psychotics, tricyclic antidepressants, MAO Inhibitors, Phenothiazines, lithium.

- Antibiotics including nitrofurantoin, erythromycin, tetracycline, gentamycin.

- Methotrexate – used to treat psoriasis and cancer

- Cimetidine - used to treat heartburn

- Salicylazosufapyridine – used to treat irritable bowel syndrome

- Phenytoin – Used in the treatment of seizures

- Sulphasalazine – Used in the treatment of ulcerative colitis

- Colchicine – Used in the treatment of gout

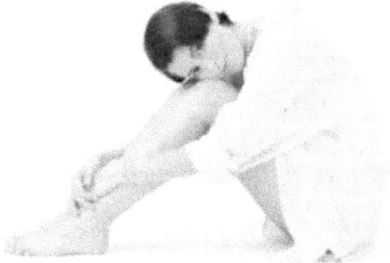

Pain Medications & Female Fertility: Some Special Advice

If you suffer from any type of chronic ache or pain – from sore, stiff knees to headaches, to monthly menstrual cramps – you may already be familiar with NSAIDs. Short for non-steroidal anti-inflammatory drugs, they include such products as aspirin and ibuprofen, and are among the most popular categories of pain relief medications in use today.

A cousin of these drugs is known as Cox2 inhibitors. They work similarly, and are also frequently prescribed to control both chronic and short term episodes of pain.

When used only occasionally or for a short period of time, there is almost no chance that these drugs will compromise your fertility – and certainly not on any kind of long term or permanent basis.

However, this can change if you use these medications on a regular basis - and particularly if you have been using them for an extended period of time.

Indeed, a number of studies have shown that NSAIDs can hamper conception by interfering with ovulation and particularly by increasing the risk of a problem known as luteinizing unruptured follicle syndrome (LUF or LUFS). In this condition, your egg follicle fails to "burst" and release an egg.

Other studies show NSAIDS may also interfere with ovulation on various other levels as well, making it much more difficult, or even impossible, to get pregnant.

In one study published in the journal *Histology and Pathology* in 2006, doctors reported that regular use of even over-the-counter NSAIDS (such as aspirin and ibuprofen) for such things as menstrual pain, could be a major contributing factor to infertility in some women – particularly in those who may already be experiencing irregular ovulation or other ovulation-related issues.

Other studies have found that even on a short term basis, ovulation can be effected for up to 7 hours after a NSAID is used. This is particularly important since many

If you are suffering severe menstrual pain, particularly pain caused by endometriosis, talk to your doctor about pain medications that won't interfere with fertility.

In addition, you can also try acupuncture . Studies show this drug-free alternative can be very helpful. Do however tell your acupuncturist that you are trying to get pregnant.

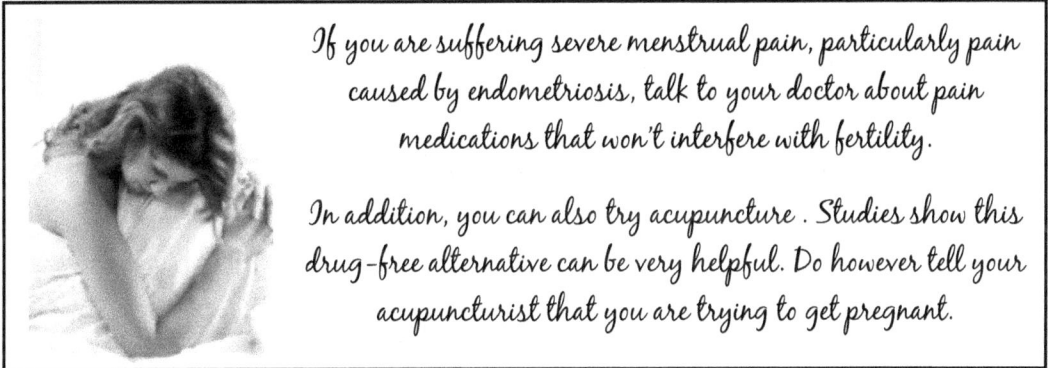

women suffer with a condition known as "Mittlesmertz" – or pain on ovulation. As a result, some doctors routinely prescribe relatively high doses of NSAIDs drugs – or recommend high doses of OTC drugs such as aspirin or ibuprofen – to be taken every few hours beginning a day or two prior to ovulation and continued until ovulation passes.

When you are not trying to conceive, this is a good pain reducing strategy. But if you are trying to get pregnant, the use of these drugs particularly in higher doses during this ovulatory time frame could definitely keep you from conceiving.

The good news: Any fertility problems related to the use of NSAIDs are completely reversible! By simply avoiding the drugs for up to 30 days prior to when you want to get pregnant (and for many women, 14 days can be adequate) you can guarantee that your system is free and clear of the effects of these medications and that your ovulation won't be affected.

If, however, you have been using these drugs regularly for an extended period of time, it may take several cycles for egg release to get back on track and normal ovulation to resume.

Remember, however, to check with your doctor before stopping any NSAIDS he or she has prescribed for a medical condition.

- **Prescription NSAIDS include**: Diclofenac, Etodolac, Fenoprofen, Flurbiprofen, Ibuprofen, Indomethacin, Meclofenamate, Mefenamic Acid, Meloxicam, Nabumetone,Naproxen, Oxaprozin, Piroxicam, Sulindac, Tolmetin

- **COX-2 inhibitors** include celecoxib.

- **Over The Counter NSAIDs include:** Aspirin, Motrin, Aleve, Advil and some menstrual pain medications.

Baby Aspirin
&
Your Baby

In addition to the research on NSAIDs and fertility, a new study published in the *Canadian Medical Association Journal* in September 2011 found that taking these drugs during the first 20 weeks of pregnancy increased the risk of miscarriage by about 35%.

As alarming as this statistic seems, many doctors believe that at least part of the problems may have been dose-related. The reason? There is also strong evidence to show that *low dose* NSAIDs, in the form of *one baby aspirin* daily, is not only safe to use while trying to conceive, but may actually help *prevent* miscarriage.

In one study which looked at 149 women enrolled in an IVF program, doctors found that one baby aspirin daily (about 80 mg of aspirin), increased ovarian responsiveness as well as increasing blood flow to the ovaries and uterus.

Not only were the women taking the baby aspirin able to make stronger and better eggs, their rate of pregnancy was nearly double that of the women who were not taking this treatment.

In addition, previous studies have shown that taking one baby aspirin a day during the first trimester may help reduce the risk of miscarriage.

So, what should you do? I frequently advised my patients at risk for miscarriage to use baby aspirin - and the results were always excellent.

But that said, if you are actively trying to conceive I suggest that you talk to your doctor about whether or not one baby aspirin a day might help encourage a faster conception.

Marijuana & Other Recreational Drugs:
What You Need To Know

It is both my recommendation and my sincere hope – that you and your partner never use any recreational drugs. First, because most of these substances can and will compromise your overall health and particularly your brain health in numerous ways. But from a strictly fertility standpoint, many recreational drugs can also dramatically impact your ability to conceive.

Indeed, one of the most commonly used recreational drugs – and one that many people falsely believe is harmless – is marijuana. Unfortunately, this is the one drug that can be exceedingly *harmful* to both male and female fertility.

In women, a number of studies have shown that marijuana can seriously impact ovulation, leading to a disruption of the menstrual cycle and compromising nearly all ovarian activity.

When *marijuana* is combined *with alcohol* – which it frequently is – the impact on fertility can be significant, even among young, otherwise healthy women.

But that's not the only problem we see. Indeed, if you should happen to get pregnant while you have marijuana and alcohol in your body, your pregnancy could end in crisis, with the combination of these drugs increasing your risk of miscarriage by over 100%.

In men, regular use of marijuana can have even more disastrous consequences, some of which are not so easy to reverse. Indeed studies show that regular use of marijuana not only reduces sperm count and semen production, but also impacts the shape and form of sperm that *is* produced. And this can dramatically affect conception.

Moreover, if your partner uses marijuana just prior to ejaculating, some of his sperm can actually get a little bit "stoned" – meaning they can't quite follow a straight path through your reproductive system to your egg. Instead they swim around in circles not really knowing where to go!

But if, in fact, they do manage to find your egg studies conducted at the University of Buffalo in New York found that compounds in marijuana inhibited the release of enzymes found in the head of the sperm, necessary to *penetrate* an egg. So, even if his sperm bumps smack into your egg, it won't matter - because no fertilization can occur unless that sperm gets inside.

While there is some evidence that stopping habitual use of marijuana will help reverse problems in some men, it does take a while. Since the active component of marijuana – a compound known as THC – is stored in fat cells, de-toxing the body isn't fast or easy. That said, the sooner he quits, the more likely it will be that his sperm count will rise and his fertility will be restored.

Cocaine and Pregnancy: Know The Facts!

Any use of cocaine – even one time – can have an overwhelming and immediate effect on your health. For some, even a one-time use can end in death. For those who do survive and continue to use this drug, there will almost assuredly be detrimental effects on fertility.The key mode of damage here is linked to the fallopian tubes, with studies showing that regular cocaine use by women can cause a type of damage that eventually destroys all chances for a natural conception.

When it comes to cocaine use, sperm can also suffer. Men who use cocaine on a regular basis are found to have reduced sperm counts, reduced sperm motility and an increased number of abnormal sperm. Moreover, if your partner has this drug in his body at the time of conception, health risks to your baby are dramatically increased. Indeed, molecules of this drug can actually attach on to the tail of sperm and literally "ride" right into an egg – so the drug and its effects are present in your baby from the moment of conception. And this, in turn can result in a number of quite serious developmental problems.

In one study published in the *Journal of the American Medical Association* (JAMA) researchers found that babies conceived by men who regularly use cocaine are much more likely to suffer serious developmental problems. In fact, the number of children born with birth defects increases in couples where one or both partners habitually use cocaine.

Steroids and Fertility: What Every Man Must Know

What's also important to note is that there is considerable evidence to show anabolic steroids (the kind used by athletes to increase muscle mass) can not only reduce sperm count, but also interfere with overall sperm production. Indeed, over the past decade we have learned much about these drugs, which include male hormones such as testosterone, as well as human growth hormone (HGH). When used correctly, under a doctor's supervision, and only when a true deficiency exists, these medications can be an important treatment. But when used without the benefit of medical supervision, and particularly when a deficiency does not exist, disastrous results can occur.

This includes testicle atrophy (meaning testicles shrink in size and begin to deteriorate), a dramatic drop in sperm count, and sometimes, complete sterility. In addition, men who use these drugs for body building purposes can also suffer an increased risk of heart problems, and experience both deep depression and excessive rage, sometimes even psychosis.

 Women who use steroid drugs to enhance athletic performance or build strength frequently find ovulation comes to a halt and their menstrual cycle stops – meaning that getting pregnant is impossible.

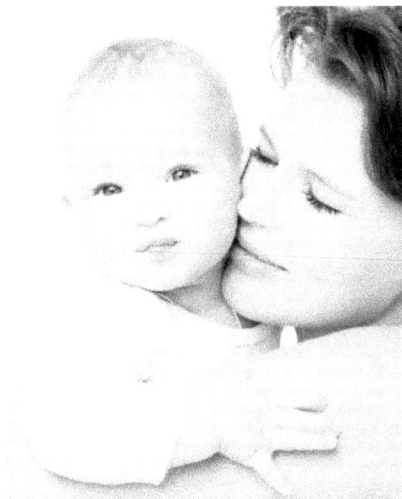

A Drug-Free Body Benefits You & Your Baby

Currently it is estimated that up to 10% of all women and men of childbearing age regularly use recreational drugs – including marijuana, cocaine or heroin, or they regularly abuse prescription drugs such as amphetamines, tranquillizers or barbiturates.

If you or your partner can count yourselves among this 10%, I hope you will heed not just these fertility warnings, but also the general health warnings that come with recreational drug use. While the reproductive risks of any drug can be based in many factors - including the substance itself and a person's individual metabolism - as a general rule I hope you will avoid the use of all recreational drugs, but particularly while you are trying to conceive.

Moreover, be aware that much of the time the impact of these substances on fertility is dose-related: The more drugs you use and the more often you use them, the greater your risks.   So while it's highly unlikely that a single dose of any drug – even a recreational one – will cause your fertility any harm, regular or habitual use can, indeed be harmful. Moreover, the younger you are when you begin drug use, the more likely it is that any damage you do sustain could become permanent.

Most Important of All: If you are trying to conceive, it is very important that you and your partner live as "clean" and as healthy a lifestyle as you possibly can. Not only will doing so help protect your general health and your fertility, but it can also help ensure that once conception does occur, your baby will have the healthiest, best start in life possible!

Remember: Healthy parents create healthy babies! Take care of yourself today and you will be helping to insure the future of all your baby's tomorrows!

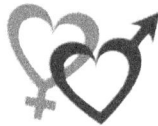

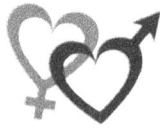

Chapter Nine

The Secrets ...

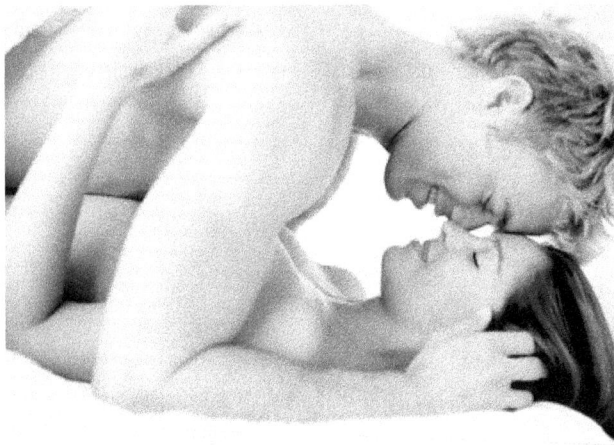

...To Making Love & Making Babies!

D o you remember the first time you and your partner laid eyes on each other? Was there magic in the air? Were sparks flying?

Or maybe when you first met, you didn't even like each other – or possibly, even despised each other ...until one day *suddenly everything changed.*

Or were you best friends for what seemed like *forever* ... and then one day turned around and realized you were in love?

Regardless of how it happens, or when it happens, or how *long it takes to happen,* once the chemistry of love is underway it's hard to imagine your life could ever have been any other way!

So what does all this have to do with getting pregnant? You might be surprised to learn that much of the very same "chemistry" that drew you and your partner together is the very same "chemistry" involved in getting pregnant! Of course this doesn't mean that you can't become pregnant when you aren't in love – of course you can. In fact, one great example of that is the use of donor sperm – where "Mom" doesn't even know "Dad's "name – and yet, pregnancy happens.

But at the same time, we also cannot deny the inexplicable role that love – as well as physical and yes sexual attraction – all play in helping to promote fertility. While this is true for both sexes, it is particularly true for women.

In fact, you may have already noticed that your attraction to your partner – and your desire for sex – increases at certain times of the month, while it dwindles or even disappears other times of the month. Of course you might think your lack of interest has mostly to do with your partner's sports-watching habits, his golf obsession , or his spending way too much time at the gym! But the truth is, your desires have less to do with your partner's comings and goings and more to do with your hormonal activity than you might realize.

Indeed, it is no coincidence of nature that as a woman approaches ovulation – a time when her body is getting ready to get pregnant – she feels more sexually stimulated and often finds her partner irresistibly more attractive during this time. Moreover, as you are about to ovulate, your cervical mucus becomes much more abundant, which also enhances sexual pleasure. So, you not only enjoy sex more during this time in your cycle, because you do, your desires also increase.

But it's not just women who feel the effects of ovulation – men sense it as well. Researchers believe that as a woman approaches ovulation, a combination of hormonal activity comes together to give off a subtle but powerful scent usually only perceived by men. When that scent is perceived it causes a quick rise in the libido and enhances his desire for sex.

Now if you're like most of my patients you may be wondering if you – or especially your partner - get these same sort of urges when either of you are around other people during "that time of the month".

In fact, I distinctly remember one patient who, after learning of these monthly biochemical signals became extremely worried that her husband may be sexually attracted to the beautiful young woman in the cubicle next to him every time that woman was ovulating!

Well the truth is chemical signals can be powerful – but love is even more powerful! Certainly, the subtle signals are always there - and in fact studies have shown that single men who meet single women for the first time find those who are ovulating more attractive.

At the same time, studies also show that when a man and woman are in a positive, loving relationship, when you are, in fact, "in love" those "outside" chemical signals are perceived far less often and to a far lesser degree than they are between partners.

In fact, when you are in a loving, supportive and caring relationship, these same chemical signals occur between partners to a much greater intensity – which is one reason why sex can be so much more fulfilling when you are in love. But it's also one of the reasons why your fertility is maximized during a loving and caring relationship.

Making Love and Making Babies: What You Must Know

When it comes to natural conception, one fact is undeniably clear: The act of making love is the optimum way of getting sperm to egg! But what many couples don't realize is that the physical chemistry involved in making love, even the mysterious mind-body interactions related to being "turned on", can also play a role in how quickly and how easily you conceive.

This is particularly true for women, since the hormonal activity that makes conception possible begins in the brain – which, not coincidentally happens to be where a woman also feels the first stirrings of sexual desire for her partner.

In fact, in order for a woman to become sexually aroused she requires not just physical stimulation, but also mental and emotional stimulation – all necessary before a truly intimate connection can be made. And it is, in fact, these mind-body connections that also play a role in fertility.

Indeed studies show that women who have a regular, satisfying sex life with intercourse at least once weekly, have more regular menstrual cycles and fewer ovulatory – related fertility problems than women whose sex life is not satisfying. But chemistry aside, it's not just hormonal activity that aligns our fertility with our sexual desires. For many couples it is also the emotional side of their relationship that can impact not just the quality of their lovemaking, but also their ability to get pregnant.

In fact, you may be surprised to learn that women who have not had a menstrual cycle for years can go into spontaneous ovulation when they fall in love! Sometimes, simply meeting "Mr. Right" can have enough of a biochemical impact to jump start hormone production and kick off ovulation in women who had met the clinical definition of "infertile" before.

Conversely, a woman who is fertile can become infertile if she is involved in a bad, abusive or otherwise negative relationship with her partner.

Getting out of that relationship and engaging with a more positive, supportive partner can often help her fertility return to normal.

Naturally, there are instances where a women becomes pregnant as a result of a rape, or even at the hands of an abusive partner - situations where there is obviously no love or support involved.

And there are also times when sperm and egg just meet – accidentally or not – and nothing will stand in the way of conception taking place.

But for many couples – and in particular for women – emotions *are* intimately entwined with reproductive biochemistry, sometimes to the point where a couples love life and the quality of their relationship can physically impact their ability to get pregnant.

Of course this does not mean to imply that all infertile couples have relationship problems. In fact, most do not.

But as you previously read, sometimes in the course of trying to get pregnant, the stress of not conceiving can begin to take its toll on a couple , often to the point where pregnancy is affected.

But in addition to the ways in which the emotional relationship between partners can impact pregnancy, so too can the physical relationship play a role - over and above having intercourse at the "right time" .

So right now I want to concentrate on the practical side of making love – and the ways in which your physical relationship with your partner can be enhanced, and in doing so help encourage your chance for getting pregnant.

The Practical Side of Sex & Fertility:

Making Love At The Right Time!

If you are like most couples trying to have a baby, you simply become "intimate" whenever the mood strikes and hope that a pregnancy happens. And while it may all seem like chance, the truth is that no matter how many times you and your partner make love, there is actually only one small window of opportunity each month when pregnancy is possible.

That "window' marks you're most fertile time frame – the interval during each monthly cycle when your egg pops from its shell, leaves your ovary and travels into your fallopian tube where it will hopefully meet up with your partner's sperm and a baby is created.

But this is more than just a "right place – right time" scenario. It is, in fact critical to the success of your conception that your egg and his sperm do "hook up" during this crucial time frame.

Why? Within 24 to 36 hours *after* your egg is ovulated it begins to disintegrate – and this means conception is not only more difficult to achieve, but when it does it may result in a defective embryo, and usually, miscarriage.

And this brings us to the first and most frequent reasons couples can't get pregnant: They make love at the wrong time!

Indeed, while most couples wait until ovulation occurs to have that critical "baby-making" sex, the truth is, by the time your egg has popped from its shell, your chance for conception drops by almost 50% - and your risk of a conceiving and then losing that conception to early miscarriage more than doubles.

In fact, many couples who believe they aren't able to get pregnant are actually conceiving – but losing that conception so early in the pregnancy, they don't even realize a pregnancy has occurred.

So when should you make love to help ensure conception takes place? The best time to start "trying" is actually up to 4 days *before* ovulation. How and why does this work? It all has to do with your partner's sperm.

Unlike your egg, which is only considered "fresh" for a short time after ovulation, the "shelf life" of your partner's sperm is a whole lot longer. In fact, from the time sperm is ejaculated into your body, it can remain alive and fully fertile for up to five days!

This means that if you begin making love two to four days *before* you expect your ovulation to occur, you and your partner will ensure there is a good supply of sperm ready and waiting for your egg to "make an entrance".

And when it does, fertilization can happen right away – when your egg is the freshest and your conception will be the healthiest.

So, how do you know two to four days before you ovulate when it's going to happen? This is where the *science* of getting pregnant comes into play.

By using easy-to-read body signs and signals, you can discover not only *when* you are *about* to ovulate, but, depending on the method you use, also get an "early warning" notice, at least four days before ovulation actually occurs.

Now, if you're like many couples you may have already tried traditional ovulation kits to help you conceive – and not had much luck. But the reason so many couples do fail to get pregnant using this technology is because no one ever told them the right way to use it.

But once you do have the secret, I can promise that you will be able to make love and make baby much quicker and easier than you think.

The Secret to Using Ovulation Prediction
to Help You Get Pregnant

As you know, ovulation is the time in your cycle when your fully matured egg pops from its shell and travels down your fallopian tube – where hopefully it will meet with your partner's sperm and fertilization will occur.   Ideally this should occur smack in the middle of your menstrual cycle. If you normally get your period every 28 days ovulation would occur on day 14; if your cycle is shorter (for example 26 days) or longer (30 or even 32 days) then ideally, the middle day of that time frame is your target ovulation date.

But that said, in today's high stress, fast paced world, it's almost impossible to find a woman who has the exact same menstrual cycle timing month in and month out. When you toss in a less-than-perfect diet, a few mild nutritional deficiencies and a bad habit or two (like smoking or drinking) you can all but toss the concept of "normal cycle" out the window!

In fact, I can tell you from my professional experience, that even young, healthy women living the perfect lifestyle don't always have completely predictable periods. Moreover, ovulation does not always occur every single month - even in young healthy women. By the time you are past age 30, you may ovulate only about 9 out of every 12 cycles – and by the time you reach age 40 you are probably ovulating less than 6 times a year.

Still, even with all these variables, I'm happy to tell you that there are a number of very reliable ways to predict when you're most fertile time will be in each and every cycle – no matter how erratic your cycles are. And that's s because all of them rely on body cues that in one way or another are linked to the hormonal activity that occurs just prior to ovulation. While the day ovulation occurs may vary from month-to-month, the biochemistry leading up to this event remains the same – which is one reason why, when used correctly, ovulation prediction can help you get pregnant!

In fact, the science of ovulation prediction was actually developed *specifically* to harness these hormonal signals and calculate them in way that helps predict when your egg is likely to pop from its shell - ripe *and ready for fertilization* – no matter when in your cycle this occurs.

But just knowing *when* you ovulate is not quite enough information to ensure a pregnancy. Indeed, as you just read, unless your timing is impeccable, waiting until the day of ovulation to be intimate with your partner can actually narrow your window of conception opportunity – particularly if his sperm is a little on the "slow" side and don't swim quite as quickly as they should.

So, the real secret to making ovulation prediction work for you: Use it to not just pinpoint your day of ovulation, but learn how to harness the power to predict, up to four days before, when ovulation is expected. Sound complicated? It's not! In fact, in the section that follows I'm going to not only teach you how to gather this valuable information - but how you and your partner can use what you learn to know exactly when to make love to make a baby.

Understanding Ovulation Prediction: Finding What Works For You!

Although the most popular form of ovulation prediction arguably comes in the form of kits found on your drugstore shelf, it's important to realize it's not the only way! There are, in fact a number of very different methods for predicting a woman's most fertile time – including some low-cost or even no-cost options.

And while the basis of all ovulation prediction methods may be somewhat the same, how each system works to detect and track this vital cycle information can be very different – which is one reason I have always advised my patients to use at least two different methods simultaneously. This will definitely help ensure the most accurate outcome.

To help you get started in choosing which of the most successful ovulation prediction methods might be right for you, I've put together the following, easy –to-use guide. It features the 5 methods I have noted as the most successful among my patients, and they also are the ways that studies show as the most accurate in predicting ovulation.

And while some of these methods are so tried-and- true they date back almost to the Bible, others are based on new inventions and discoveries – and some even rely on the latest high tech electronics. That said. don't be fooled into thinking that *newer* is always *better*. Most of the time, newer is just, well, *newer.* So in this respect you should simply choose the methods that seem easiest, most convenient and most cost - effective *for you.*

I do, however, have one final piece of advice: Please keep in mind that ovulation prediction systems can only reflect what is already going on in your body. If there is a problem within your reproductive system – from physical issues such as blocked fallopian tube from endometriosis or a sexually transmitted infection or if hormonal problems are preventing ovulation - an ovulation prediction system isn't a cure, and it isn't a way around these problems.

At the same time however, if a problem does exist, many of these ovulation prediction methods can also provide you with some important information about why a pregnancy might not be happening - data that together with your doctor you can look at, analyze, and in many instances, do something about. For many, the solution may require nothing more than the suggestions you will find in this book, regarding diet and lifestyle changes.

In fact, as you begin to chart your ovulation schedule, it's also important that you simultaneously begin to implement at least some of the suggestions found throughout this book. Together with knowing the "right" time to get pregnant, you'll have the "one-two punch" that will significantly boost your odds of conception!

Ovulation Prediction Method # 1: The BBT
Using Your Body Temperature To Help You Get Pregnant

In the classic situation comedy, attempts at getting pregnant are often portrayed by a wife making a frantic call to her hubby whispering that her temperature is "up" – and it's time to make love! Inevitably he's at the gym, in a business meeting, or about to board a plane when the call comes – and the comedy takes flight as he jumps through hoops to make it home "in time".

And while this scenario is rooted in some truth – body temperature does rise and fall in relation to ovulation – the fact is that once your body temperature rises, ovulation has already passed.

So unless your partner is "ready, willing and able "at the exact moment your temperature rises, this is not the "signal" you should be looking for.

So what temperature related sign should you is watching for? A subtle but important *drop* that occurs just before ovulation is about to take place.

Indeed, during your entire menstrual cycle – and especially in the days leading up to ovulation - your body undergoes a series of hormonal fluctuations, at least some of which influence what is called your **Basal Body Temperature or BBT.** This represents the measurement of your "core" body temperature while you are at rest. By taking your BBT every day, starting on the first day of your menstrual cycle, you'll be able to see when the subtle drop occurs. When it does you'll know that ovulation is likely to follow within 12 to 24 hours.

Once ovulation has occurred, you'll get a subtle rise in body temperature – usually about ½ a degree. At this point you'll know that your chances for getting pregnant are about to decline, and will do so rapidly over the next 12 to 24 hours.

TO GET PREGNANT FAST: Begin making love the moment your temperature drops (around mid-cycle) and continue being intimate with your partner as often as you like until 24 hours after your temperature rises again.

An Alternate Method: If you chart your BBT everyday for two to three months, you will begin to see a pattern emerge – one that allows you to "predict" when the drop in temperature is going to occur. With this information you and your partner can begin to make love every day, beginning 3 to 5 days *before* you expect the temperature drop. You should continue making love until your temperature rises again.   Because, as you just learned, sperm can live in a woman's body for up to five days, making love prior to ovulation means you will have plenty of sperm ready and waiting in your fallopian tube the minute your egg "arrives". This is the fastest and the best way to insure a pregnancy will occur

Some Extra BBT Success Tips

1.   **Establish a BBT Schedule**
As easy as the BBT method is to use, it's important to note that other factors besides ovulation can alter body temperature. A lack of sleep, for example, as well as stress, diet, even a slight cold or virus can all force changes in your BBT. For this reason you should begin charting your BBT at least two months prior to when you want to get pregnant and again, look for the pattern to emerge.

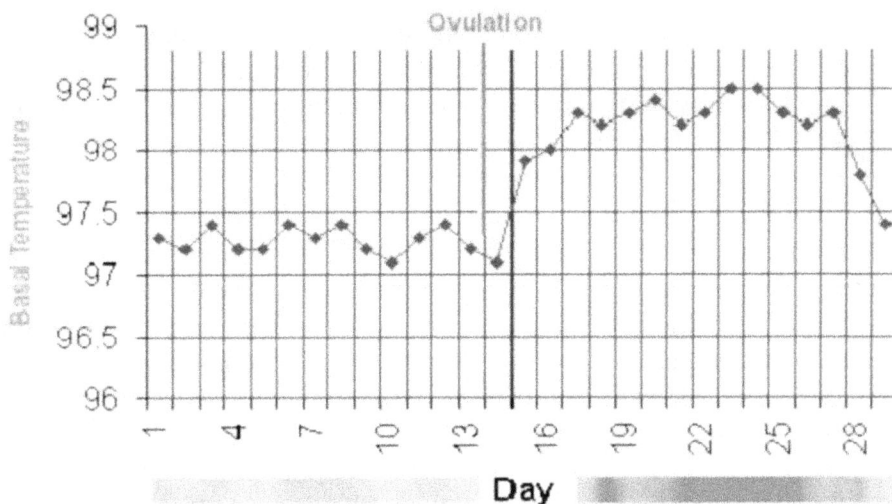

To get pregnant fast: Make love when your temperature drops and before it rises - this coincides with the timing of your ovulation.

2. Be Timely!

To get the most reliable BBT readings possible – and to accurately predict when ovulation is about to occur – take your temperature at the same time every day.   The best time is first thing in the morning, before getting out of bed, eating or drinking anything and certainly before smoking - though it is my hope that you will have stopped by this time. This will help ensure it is your *true* BBT – and that in turn will make it easier to predict ovulation.

3.   Use a BBT Thermometer

While it's not critical to use a BBT thermometer, doing so can help ensure a more accurate temperature reading. Why? A BBT thermometer is more sensitive, so it is capable of alerting you to small changes in your body temperature that might otherwise go unnoticed. Indeed, while some women see an obvious drop in temperature right before ovulation – one-half to one degree – for some the change can be more subtle, and might easily go unregistered on a regular thermometer.   While a good BBT thermometer can cost a bit more, if you shop around you should be able to get one at a good price - and I believe its well worth a few extra dollars.

4. Write It Down!

While you might think it's simple to remember temperature changes – and that it's easy to note when the drop occurs – still, it's very helpful to keep a written daily record. Moreover, remember that part of your goal should be to establish a temperature *pattern*, which is far easier to see when you are looking at a written chart.

While you certainly can keep track of your temperature in any notebook, most of my patients found it much easier to use a pre-made BBT chart – like the one pictured on the previous page. As you can see the chart not only makes it easy to record numbers, but when you "connect the dots" it also gives you an excellent graphic representation of when your body temperature changes. A side-by-side comparison of your monthly charts can also make it super easy to track ovulation and predict when the time is right to make love. You can download a free BBT blank chart at: http://www.gettingpregnantnow.org/articles/ovulation-bbt-guide.html On the same page, you can also download a free Ovulation EBook guide that explains all your options more fully.

Ovulation Prediction Method # 2: Listen To Your Body

In addition to temperature changes, there is another way your body lets you know that ovulation is approaching. And it's through changes in your cervical mucus and in the shape of your cervix. While this may sound like signs only your doctor could recognize, it's actually quite easy for you to determine on your own.

What can make it even easier is to do your first "cervical check up" as soon as your menstrual cycle ends. Because this is a time when we know for certain you cannot get pregnant, it will allow you to establish an important "base line" reading. So, later in your cycle, as ovulation approaches, you'll have something to compare your body signs and signals to.

Here's how to do your first cervical mucus/ cervical shape test:

1. Begin by washing your hands thoroughly with soap and warm water.
2. Separate the outside lips of your vulva and gently insert your finger into your vagina. You should be able to feel your cervical mucus. Take note of how it feels. If you taking this test at the beginning of your cycle your mucous should feel somewhat dry.

3. Insert your finger just a little farther in, until you feel your cervix. Again, if this is at the start of your cycle, it should be in a "low" position, slightly pointy and hard, and relatively easy to feel.

Now that you know where to look, and what to look for - you can use this information to track and follow the changes in both the shape and feel of your cervix and the consistency of your cervical mucus – both of which undergo some specific changes as your body approaches ovulation.

To help you track those changes, here is a short guide on what to look for throughout a single cycle.

Stage One: As a Menstrual Cycle Ends
Mucous: At the end of your cycle, your vagina should feel somewhat dry – in fact, for some of you it may feel so dry that you don't feel any mucous at all.

Corresponding Cervical Changes: During and right after menstruation your cervix will be in a low position. It will be easy to touch and it will feel firm and have a somewhat pointy shape. You should have no problems locating or feeling it.

Stage Two: One-Third into a New Cycle
Mucous: About a third of the way into a new cycle – about the 9th or 10th day after your last period ended your mucous will take on a creamy wet look and feel. It will seem somewhat thicker than before, and should be fairly abundant.

Corresponding Cervical Changes: Your cervix may feel as if it's "receding "or pulling up inside your body, which, in fact, is the case. You may have to reach a little deeper inside to touch it, but when you do it will still feel somewhat firm.

Stage Three: Mid-Cycle, Approaching Ovulation
Mucous: Regardless of the length of your cycle, as you approach the mid-point, your mucous will begin to feel thin and slippery and have a somewhat "stretchy" consistency. By the time you actually reach ovulation, it will resemble raw egg white: Almost translucent, and with a more liquid look and feel. This occurs in order to facilitate the transport of sperm through your vaginal canal and into your fallopian tube. Indeed, one very common cause of infertility is mucous that does not become thin enough at the time of ovulation to successfully transport sperm (see: When Sperm Is Stuck on the next page)

Corresponding Cervical Changes: As your body responds to an increase in estrogen, your cervix pulls up slightly, and rotates forward, making it easier for your partner's sperm to reach your egg. At the same time, however, it makes it a little more difficult for you to touch your cervix – which is actually a sign that ovulation is approaching. If you do feel it, you'll notice that it seems softer to the touch and somewhat wetter. This is because at this point in your cycle your mucous is very abundant, creating a soft "wet" feeling inside.

Infertile		You Can Get Pregnant		Infertile	
			Open	Closed	
Your Cycle Begins	Mucous Is Thick	Mucous Begins To Thin	Mucous Is Very Thin	Mucous Begins To Thicken	Mucous Is Once Again Thick

Stage Four: After Ovulation Occurs

Mucous: Unless fertilization occurs, within hours after you ovulate your mucous supply begins to dwindle.   Within 24 to 36 hours after ovulation, your mucous production takes a sharp decline. Whatever is left becomes extremely thick and sticky, with an almost glue-like consistency.   Many women have reported it looks and feels somewhat like rubber cement!   Generally speaking, your mucous will remain this way for two to three days, after which time it often becomes so dry you can barely feel it. And in fact, it's not usual for sex to feel uncomfortable during this time, simply because of the lack of lubrication. Of course when you are sexually stimulated you will produce some mucous, but it will be nowhere near the quantity that is present around the time of ovulation.

Corresponding Cervical Changes: As your mucous is drying, your cervix responds by dropping back down, once again making it easier to touch. It will also feel harder and firmer again, much like it did at the start of your cycle.   This is caused by a drop in estrogen levels.

TO GET PREGNANT FAST: Using your mucous production and cervical changes as a guide, the easiest way to insure a quick pregnancy is to begin making love at **Stage Two** when your mucous is creamy and wet - which occurs 3 to 4 days prior to ovulation.   Remember, your partner's sperm can live in your body for up to 5 days, so starting early can insure that you won't miss the chance to have sperm ready and waiting when ovulation does occur.

To ensure your chances even more, continue being intimate with your partner until you see a noticeable decline in mucous production. This, of course, signals that ovulation has occurred, and it is highly unlikely that you will conceive.

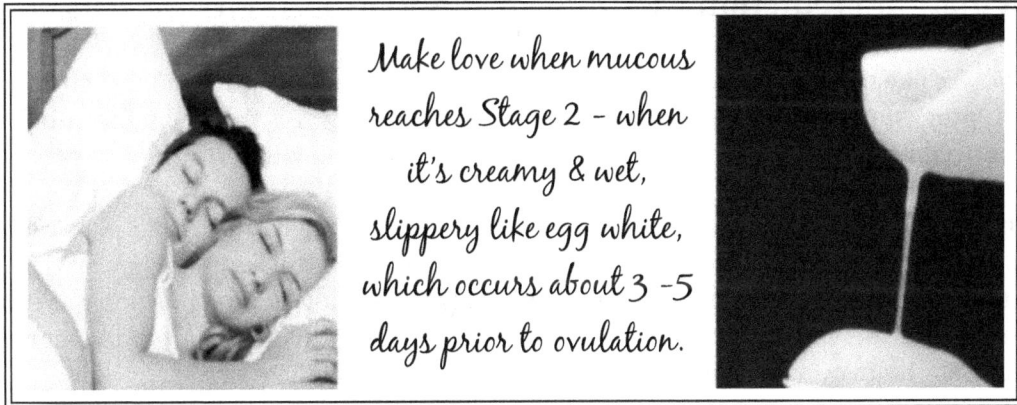

Make love when mucous reaches Stage 2 - when it's creamy & wet, slippery like egg white, which occurs about 3 -5 days prior to ovulation.

When Sperm Gets Stuck: What to Do

One of the leading "hidden" causes of infertility is also one of the simplest to treat. It occurs when your mucous is simply too thick to allow your partner's sperm to swim through your reproductive system and reach your egg on time! Indeed, when this occurs, sperm can actually get "stuck" midstream – and not be able to move! Even if your mucous is only slightly thicker than normal, if your partner's sperm are slightly defective, with a reduced ability to swim, problems can also occur.

In either scenario taking steps to thin your mucous will help your partner's sperm move more freely and reach your egg faster and easier. So how do you do this?

One way is for you to avoid whole fat dairy products, including milk, ice cream and yogurt during this time, since these foods can cause mucus to thicken. If you cut these out of your diet beginning at the start of your menstrual cycle you may find that you are producing what seems like more abundant mucus, but what is actually just thinner mucus – which is much more advantageous to getting pregnancy.

Another way, is to thin your mucus by taking a cough medicine containing the ingredient guaifenesin. Much the way it thins the mucous in your lungs when you have congestion, guaifenesin will also thin the mucous in your reproductive system. Be certain however the cough medicine contains only guaifenesin – such as *Robitussin for Chest Congestion*. If the cough medicine also contains the cough suppressant dextromethorphan don't use it. There are some reports this ingredient may interfere with a healthy conception.

Ovulation Prediction Method # 3: Ovulation Predictor Kits

If you're like most of my patients, then you probably associate the hormones estrogen and progesterone with getting pregnant. And indeed, as the main hormones produced by your reproductive system, they are indeed key to fertility.

But as you read earlier, neither estrogen nor progesterone can begin to play their respective roles until well after two other hormones are in full swing. They are FSH (short for follicle stimulating hormone) and LH (short for luteinizing hormone). Both are secreted by your brain, and without them your eggs would not get the signal necessary to grow and develop, and ovulation could not take place.

As you read earlier, FSH jump-starts the baby-making process by sending a chemical message to your ovaries to begin turning your egg follicles into actual eggs. When one reaches maturity, estrogen levels are peaking – which in turn tells your brain it's time to release LH, the hormone which prompts your ovary to release your egg so that ovulation can occur. In fact, normally within 24 hours after the surge of LH, your egg will pop from its shell and swim into your fallopian tube to meet up with your partner's sperm.

And it is *this* activity that allows ovulation prediction kits to work! How? Once your LH surges, it's quickly processed by your body, causing the natural chemical residues to be discharged into your urine. Ovulation prediction kits work by measuring the LH residue in your urine. Using test strips chemically treated to register these residues, an ovulation prediction kit tells you when LH has been secreted – which is the signal that ovulation *is about to occur.*

TO GET PREGNANT FAST:
By urinating on the test strips once daily, beginning around the 9th day of your cycle, you can watch for your LH surge color change. Once you see it, you know ovulation is eminent, and will usually occur within 24 hours or less. So, one way to insure a pregnancy is to begin making love as soon as the test strip indicates the presence of LH.   Continue making love any time the mood strikes you, for up to 48 hours afterwards.

To Dramatically Increase Your Success: Begin using the ovulation prediction kit a few months *prior* to when you want to get pregnant. Using the blank chart from the Basal Body Temperature or BBT guide, indicate the start of your cycle, when you start testing, and when the LH surge appears on your test strip. Do this every month for two or three months, after which time you will see a pattern start to emerge – one that indicates the days in your cycle when you are most likely to *expect ovulation*. The month you want to get pregnant, begin making love 3 to 5 days prior to when you *expect* ovulation to occur. Continue to use the test strip during this time, and continue being intimate with your partner while the test strip is registering that ovulation is approaching.   This will help ensure there is sperm ready and waiting when ovulation does occur.

If you use an ovulation predictor kit in conjunction with either your BBT or your Body Signs, then your chances of getting pregnant will increase even more.

Ovulation Prediction Method # 4: The Saliva Test

One of the newer – and some say more reliable – ways to predict not only ovulation, but a variety of hormonal activity linked to conception, is through the analysis of saliva. How is this possible?

Research shows that many of the hormonal changes that occur just prior to ovulation yield corresponding changes in saliva!   By tracking those changes you can predict when ovulation will occur.

While this may sound like a high school "science experiment". the truth is, the method is simple and the test kits that help you do this are quick and easy to use.

How the Saliva Test Works
You begin by placing a drop of saliva on a glass slide (included with the test kit), and letting it dry – which should take 10 minutes or less.   When saliva dries, the liquid portion crystallizes into various patterns called "ferns" – because they, in fact, do resemble ferns. These formations occur in direct response to hormonal levels – and the shape goes through some distinct changes in relation to hormonal fluctuations that occur just prior to ovulation.

While you can't see these changes in your saliva with the naked eye, by viewing tiny droplets under a microscope (included in the test kit) these changes do become easily apparent.

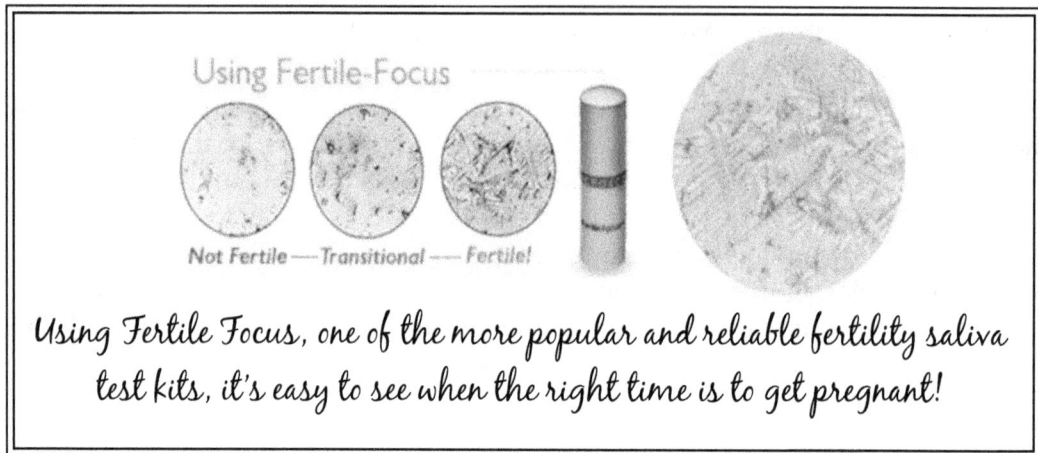

Using Fertile Focus, one of the more popular and reliable fertility saliva test kits, it's easy to see when the right time is to get pregnant!

In fact, each kit comes with an inexpensive but powerful portable microscope (about the size of a lipstick tube) that is specifically designed to not just magnify what you see, but actually enhance and define the crystallization process of saliva.

By placing the hand held microscope over the glass slide containing your saliva, you will be able to quickly and easily view the crystallized patterns.

If you begin viewing your saliva at the start of your cycle, and you continue to view it every day, somewhere around the 9th day you will see the fern pattern begin to take shape. This is an indication that ovulation is 3 to 5 days away.

TO GET PREGNANT FAST: Begin making love as soon as you notice a change in your saliva crystal pattern.

While you should see the "fern" shape start to form beginning around day 9 of your cycle, in some women, that shape is not quite clear. If this is the case, just look for *any change in shape*. Most of the time this will be indicative of the hormonal activity that signals ovulation time is near.

You should continue making love daily for up to 7 days after you see the change.

The Ova Cue Saliva Testing PLUS!

If you want to take your ovulation prediction into the computer age, then the OvaCue is for you! This ingenious little hand-held computer uses a spoon-sized electronic sensor to "read" the hormonal changes in saliva. You simply place the sensor on your tongue for five seconds every morning, and OvaCue will automatically display your "fertility status" for that day. A tiny built-in "ova –brain" tracks the readings and holds them in the memory. As you approach your most fertile time the computer indicates when you should start trying to get pregnant! Plus, OvaCue also comes with software that allows you to download your readings directly into your computer or smart phone and track them on a calendar.

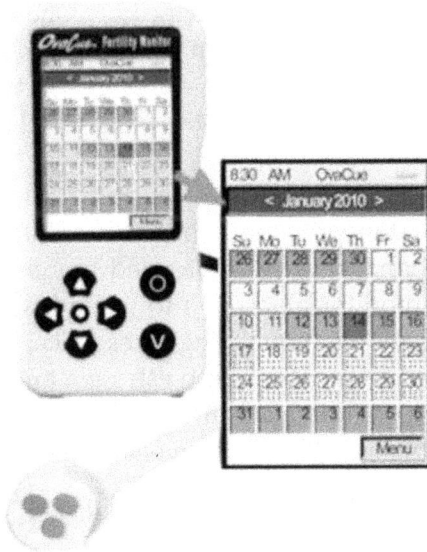

But how reliable is the Ova-Cue? Independent studies published in over 10 top medical journals have not only proven that OvaCue works, but that it is among the most effective methods available to predict ovulation up to a full seven days before it happens!

Ovulation Prediction Method # 5: Fertility Monitors

In many respects, every type of ovulation prediction method mentioned in this chapter is a type of "fertility monitor". In fact, any test which helps alert you to the time frame preceding ovulation is, in a sense, monitoring your fertility.

But that said, in recent years a bumper crop of new test kits known specifically as "fertility monitors" have burst on the scene. Although each one functions slightly differently, they all have one goal in common: To help determine when you are going to ovulate.

So, how is this different from other types of ovulation predictor kits or methods? Primarily the difference is in the time frame and the amount of advance notification

Primarily the difference is in the time frame and the amount of advance notification these kits can provide. How do they do it? Much like ovulation predictor kits, fertility monitors rely on hormone levels found in urine. But where they differ is in the hormones that are measured.

I explained earlier how an ovulation prediction kit measures LH – the hormone that is secreted 12 to 14 hours before ovulation occur. A fertility monitor measures not only LH, but also estrogen levels leading up to the surge in LH – and that in turn gives you the opportunity to "predict" ovulation with advance notice of up to 7 days.

In the Clear-Blue Easy Fertility Monitor pictured below - one the most popular brands sold today – testing is actually a two step process. It begins by entering personal information about your cycle into a hand held computerized monitoring device. Using this information as a guide the monitor alerts you to when it's time to begin step two , which is when the actual hormonal monitoring takes place. This step utilizes chemically sensitive strips designed to measure both estrogen and LH residues in urine. The results of each test strip reading are also entered into the monitoring device which calculates three sub-cycles within each menstrual cycle.

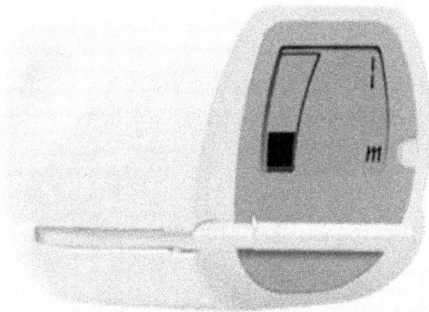

The 3 Sub-Cycles Are As Follows:

Low - The chance of conception is very small - not impossible, but almost!

High - There is a chance for conception with this phase, typically representing about 5 days prior to ovulation

Peak: This is the time frame just prior to ovulation and represents the highest chance of conception immediately following intercourse.

TO GET PREGNANT FAST: Begin making love when your fertility monitor indicates you are in "**HIGH**" conception status. Continue having regular intercourse at least once daily until you are 24 hours past the time when your fertility monitor registers "**PEAK**" conception status.

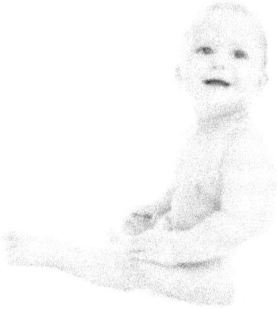

Ovulation Prediction:
Some Final Advice

Certainly the "science "of ovulation prediction is not as precise as we would like it to be. In addition to all of the factors that can influence the tests themselves, many more factors can influence ovulation – to the point where month to month changes can make it difficult and frustrating for some women to predict their most fertile time.

If this turns out to be the case for you, don't stress over it – and don't worry. Just use these methods to the best of your ability.   If you pay attention to the signs I promise you will garner some important information that will help you get pregnant – or at least better understand the reasons why you are having difficulty.

Moreover when you combine the information you glean from ovulation prediction, with the additional hints and tips found in the next two chapters, and the nutritional and lifestyle information found throughout the book, all the pieces of your personal fertility puzzle will begin to fit together in a way that increases your chances of getting pregnant.

 For most of you this information will be more than enough to insure you get pregnant – and to do so faster and easier. For the few who may still have problems, having as much information as you can about how your body functions will ultimately help your doctor to better *help you* and your partner select the treatment options that will yield

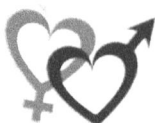

Chapter Ten

Your Complete Guide
To Baby-Making Sex!

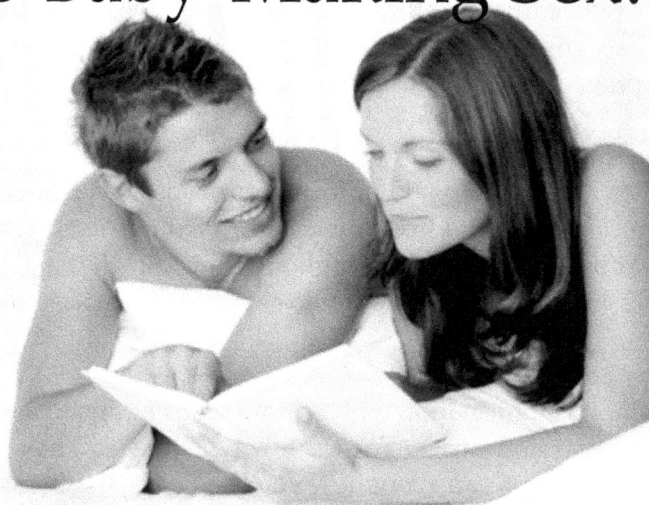

The Secrets Every Couple Must Know!

W hen it comes to making love, I'm pretty confident that each of you are doing just fine on your own!

Indeed, as an expression of the intimacy and emotional connection between you and your partner, you may have already figured out sex can often be the "glue" that helps bind together all aspects of your relationship. In fact, studies show that couples who "bond" together sexually often have a better relationship overall, both in and out of bed.

That said, it's also important to remember that "great sex" is subject to highly personal interpretation. Indeed, what can seem "wild and fabulous" to one couple may seem "boring and tame" to another. Likewise, what's acceptable in one bedroom may not be acceptable in the bedroom next door.

Hopefully you and your partner have found not just a level of sexual compatibility but also sexual intimacy, a place where you both feel safe, satisfied and happy and your relationship feels complete.

So what does all this have to do with "baby making sex"? Well, for some couples, nothing! Indeed, I'm sure you know of many couples who just stop birth control and continue on with their normal sex life, and are pregnant within a month or two. In fact, nothing about how or even when they have sex seems to matter - pregnancy just happens!

For some, however, particularly those of you for whom pregnancy is taking longer than expected, everything about "baby making sex" can take on a new and different meaning. Suddenly it's not just about "making love" any more, it's about "making a baby" and with that change can come some major changes in how you and your partner relate not just to sex, but to each other.

For those struggling month after month to get pregnant – and particularly if you are taking fertility medications to help you conceive – then "sex on demand" becomes a new part of your intimate vocabulary, and in the process can complicate or even totally upset what might have been a perfectly delightful sex life before!

In fact, it is not at all uncommon for many couples to feel so much pressure about having sex at the "right time", that they lose much of the fun and the passion, the intimacy and the enjoyment that was such a great part of their sex life before.

Well if any of this is true for you, I have some great news to share. Because what you are going to learn in this chapter are not only some great tips and important advice on how to turn a your sex life into exciting "baby making" sex, but also how to keep the love and the fun and the sheer joy of your intimate life at the center of your pregnancy goals .

While not every piece of the advice or every suggestion in this section will apply to all couples, I do invite you to read all of it with an open mind and an open heart – and to share this chapter with your partner. If you work together, I promise that you can turn your baby making sex into not only one of the most pleasurable times of your life, but also one of the most memorable. And why shouldn't it be? These are the times when you are creating a brand new life – and nothing is more memorable or more spectacular or more romantic than that!

Having Sex – Making Babies: How to Make It Happen Faster

As I mentioned at the very start of this chapter, for some lucky couples simply making love when the mood strikes is enough to ensure pregnancy. But for far more couples – and particularly for those who aren't getting pregnant right away - this isn't the case. Try as they might, pregnancy doesn't seem to happen.

Of course sometimes there is a medical or hormonal problem that is blocking conception. But what many otherwise normal, healthy couples don't realize is that when it comes to making babies, *how* you make love can be as important as *when you make love.*

Indeed, the operative function here is getting sperm to egg – so in many respects as long as intercourse occurs within 5 days prior to and during ovulation there's a good possibility this is going to happen.

That said, there are also a number of what I like to call "intimacy variables" – ways of making love that can definitely influence how quickly you get pregnant!

So what are the best ways to make love – and have a baby?

1. Male Dominant or "missionary" position. While it may not be the most exciting way to make love, when it comes to getting pregnant, "man on top" has some definite advantages – not the least of which is a clear path to "shooting" sperm deep into the vagina.

This position can be made even more effective if you place a pillow under your pelvic region, causing your vagina to be tilted slightly more backwards. Again, this will help facilitate the flow of sperm into your reproductive tract, and also help avoid "back ward flow "– a situation where sperm which may not be the best swimmers actually take a retrograde path out of the vagina.

2. **Knee-To-Chest or "rear entry" position -** Using this technique you bring your knees very close to your chest while your partner slips inside your vagina from underneath. This position allows your partner to deposit his sperm much deeper, and much closer to your cervix, meaning many more sperm are likely to make their way inside. This can be an especially good position if your partner has a marginally low or even very low sperm count. The increase in pregnancy success can be dramatic!

3. **Lying on your side** - This position can very conducive to pregnancy if either you or your partner suffer from any back pain, or if either of you is over-weight. By taking pressure off the nerves in the lower portion of your pelvis you may be able to relax more and this could influence how quickly and easily sperm can make their way to your fallopian tube.

The WORST Love Making Positions for Getting Pregnant: Sitting, standing and female dominant (woman on top).

All these positions slow down the transport of sperm and can make conception more difficult.

Can Wild Energetic Sex Help You Get Pregnant?

While it's clear that sexual positions make a difference, a bold new suggestion from a group of British fertility experts suggests that the "wilder" and more "energetic" the sex is, the greater the chance for getting pregnant!

Indeed, many experts now believe that if you can recreate the earliest, most erotic days of your relationship in your marital bed right now, the better your chances are for conceiving. What's the connection?

One reason has to do with sperm. Most average, healthy men eject about 250 million sperm during each ejaculation. But studies show that men who are fully aroused and enjoying optimal sexual stimulation actually eject about 50% more sperm – thus increasing the chance of conception by a significant margin. Indeed what many men do not realize is that the more excited they are during sex, the further back into the testicle the body reaches to pull out more sperm – and that dramatically increases the pregnancy power of each ejaculation.

According to British fertility researcher Dr. Allan Pacey at Sheffield University, as little as 5 extra minutes of exciting sexual activity prior to ejaculation can mean an extra 25 million sperm are available for conception. Moreover, these extra sperm appear of be of higher quality than normal, average sperm, which further helps increase not just the chance for pregnancy but also that the conception will be a healthy one.

This research dovetails perfectly with previous studies showing that men who view pornography just prior to ejaculating are able to put out much greater amounts of sperm. In fact, one reason many fertility clinics provide sexually exciting materials for men to read prior to giving an insemination sperm sample, is so the highest concentration of good sperm becomes readily available.

Women, Wild Sex and Getting Pregnant: How Orgasm Can Help

In case you're wondering if it's just male fertility that benefits from super exciting sex, the truth is, female fertility may also gain some benefits. Indeed, studies show that more female orgasms don't just lead to more enjoyable sex, they can also lead to enhanced fertility. How?

During an orgasm, the intense muscle contractions occurring within the entire pelvic region cause a kind of pressure to develop in and around the uterus. Many experts believe that this pressure acts as a kind of "sexual vacuum" literally sucking the sperm more deeply into the cervix and eventually, into the uterus itself.

Indeed, in one study which measured the "flow back" of sperm that leaked out of a woman's body after sex, researchers found that women who had an orgasm a minute or less before their partner ejaculated retained far more sperm than women who either didn't have an orgasm or who had one much earlier than their partners.

Interestingly the study also found that if a woman had an orgasm up to 45 minutes after her partner ejaculated, sperm retention was higher than if she had no orgasm.

Moreover, because an orgasm can help you feel relaxed and even sleepy, many believe this increases your pregnancy odds by encouraging you to lie still after sex – which is still another way to encourage conception (See page 250).

YOUR GUIDE TO BABY-MAKING SEX

Morning Sex vs. Night Sex: Which Is Better?

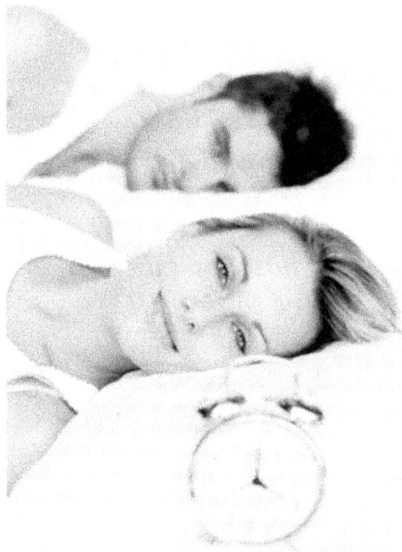

Q: *I've heard that it's easier to get pregnant if you have sex in the morning. Is this true?*

A: Many couples have asked me whether or not the time of day they make love can influence the ease with which they conceive. And the answer is "No" – with some qualifying information.

While there are no studies to show that the rate of pregnancy is influenced by the time of day a couple makes love, these odds *could* change if your partner has even a marginally low sperm count. Why?

Generally speaking, a man's hormones are at their peak in the morning upon waking – one reason why many men are more sexually stimulated at this time then they are at night. But besides the issue of desire, there is also evidence that sperm count may be higher in the mornings as well. So, if it's enjoyable for both of you, you can maximize his sperm potential by making love after a good night's rest. It just might help you get pregnant faster!

Moreover, with most couples leading such busy, hectic lives - with women in particular being pulled in so many different directions - making love in the morning, when both you and your partner are more rested can encourage reproductive hormone activity essential for getting pregnant.

Indeed, as you learned earlier in this book, stress – and the hormones produced by the body's response to stress – are virtual "fertility killers".

Moreover sleep is one of the most powerful antidotes to stress, which not only helps reduce the production of nasty compounds manufactured when you are under stress, but also helps mediate some important fertility chemicals as well. So, if you and your

Lying Still After Sex?

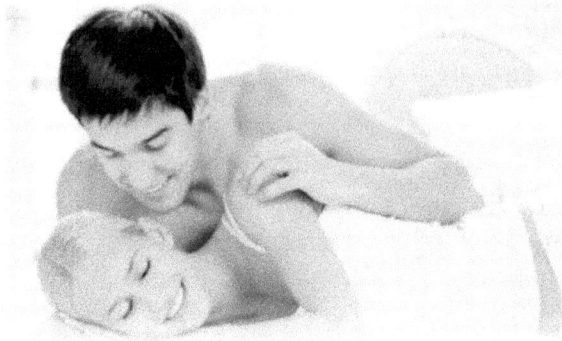

Q: *Someone told me that if you lie still after sex it's easier for conception to occur . Is this true?*

If so, how long do you have to lie still?

A: Among the many questions I receive from patients about boosting conception odds, by far the most popular involves whether or not lying still after sex – and not jumping from the bed - can help. And I believe that it can.

In fact, one of the very earliest medical theories about links between female orgasm and increased fertility was called the "Poleaxes" hypothesis. And it stated that because following orgasm most women feel relaxed and somewhat sleepy, most tend to lie down and take a nap after sex – which many doctors believed help increase the chance that sperm would remain in her body longer and thus increase the chance for pregnancy to occur.

As you just read, we now have an updated and far more logical reason why orgasm increases fertility.

But this doesn't negate the fact that lying down after sex might help.

Indeed, in one study conducted on women undergoing IUI (intra-uterine insemination) it was learned that those who remained in a horizontal position after the procedure for just 15 minutes were almost twice as likely to get pregnant than those who jumped up and began moving about shortly thereafter.

In fact, while it takes sperm anywhere from two to ten minutes to reach the fallopian tube following ejaculation, there's no guarantee that "contact" will be made in that specific time frame - even if your egg is ready and waiting! So in this instance, lying down after sex can help insure that his sperm is given the best possible opportunity to travel through your uterus and into your fallopian tube and connect with your egg.

Moreover, if you follow the ovulation prediction guidelines in the previous chapter and begin to have sex 3 to 4 days prior to your expected time of egg release, lying in bed after sex can really give you a distinct pregnancy advantage. Because your partner's sperm will literally be "parked" in your uterus and tubes waiting for your egg to arrive, the more you can control the backward flow out of your reproductive system, the higher the concentration of sperm will be when you finally do ovulate.

How Much Sex Is Too Much Sex?

When it comes to the amount of sex necessary for getting pregnant, as the old saying goes, it can happen on the very first try! And for some couples it does.

For most, however, it's going to take more than one night of sexy fun to make a baby.

While in the past it was believed that having sex too often can drain a man's sperm resources and actually reduce the chance for conception, you and your partner may be happy to learn that if he is healthy, you can have as much sex as you want and sperm won't be affected.

In fact, one interesting new study revealed that the men who may benefit most from frequent ejaculations include those with a higher-than-normal level of "abnormal" sperm, or those with a partner who has a history of 'unexplained' recurring miscarriage. hy? It seems that frequent ejaculations actually *reduce* the amount of abnormal sperm present in any given pregnancy attempt.

As explained in research presented recently at the annual European Society of Human Reproduction and Embryology by Dr. David Greening of Sydney IVF in Australia, after daily ejaculations for 7 days straight, 81% of the men showed a marked *decrease* in DNA-damaged sperm. Frequent ejaculations were also linked to a slight increase in sperm motility – perhaps because there were a higher percentage of normal, healthy sperm on the job!

While doctors aren't certain as to why the sperm seemed healthier and speedier after frequent ejaculations, Dr. Greening speculates it could be that sperm which is ejaculated soon after being made may be "fresher" than the sperm which sits in the reproductive system for days before being ejaculated.

Certainly if your partner's sperm count is even marginally low I would recommend that he abstain from ejaculating for a few days prior to when you want to start conceiving.

Moreover, even if his sperm count and sperm health is normal – and you have no history of miscarriage, it is my personal belief that abstaining from ejaculation for two to three days prior to when you want to start conceiving, is still a good idea.   If you do this, then you can feel very comfortable about having sex every day or even several times a day during your most fertile time. And this, I believe is the best way to dramatically increase your pregnancy odds.

The "Scent" of Fertility:
A Natural Sexy Way To Encourage Conception

Have you ever noticed that you like the way your partner smells? I don't mean his aftershave or cologne or shower gel – I mean the way *he* smells when he isn't wearing any fragrance of any kind. Or maybe you simply like being around him – and never even noticed that it's his personal fragrance that makes being with him feel so good.

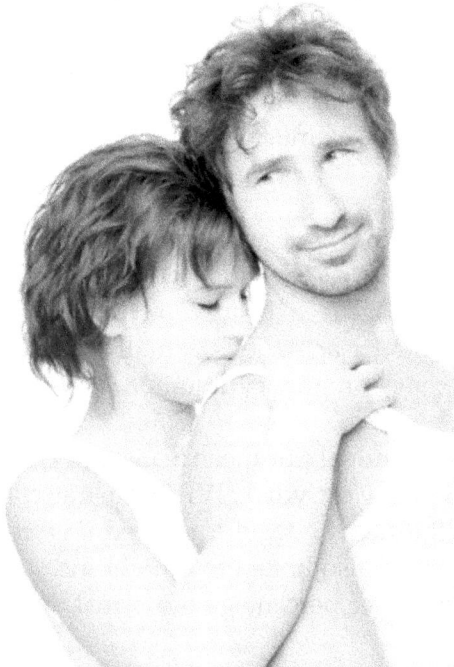

Whether you have noticed his scent – or you haven't - the truth is that both you and your partner give off a subtle unique odor based on the production of what are known as "pheromones". These are hormones that, among other things, are designed to give off silent signals that attract us to our mate. In fact, some research shows that using our sense of smell we unconsciously seek out someone with whom our DNA will be a perfect blend so that we *can* make healthy babies!

Moreover studies published in the journal *Nature* and other publications have shown that certain partner scents can encourage ovulation, even in women who are having problems making eggs! Indeed, studies show that the scent of a man's perspiration when he is turned on is not only able to turn on a woman, but, over time, increases her fertility by helping to regulate her menstrual cycles. In reports presented to the American Chemical Society by the Monsell Chemical Senses Center in Philadelphia, it has been suggested that these natural odors influence the secretion of a variety of hormones linked to fertility.

In addition, as I mentioned earlier, studies show many men can actually "smell" when a woman is ovulating, and feel more sexually attracted to her during this time. In studies conducted at Florida State University researchers found that men who smelled the T-shirts of women who were ovulating experienced a wild surge in testosterone – which as you probably know is the hormone responsible for a man's sex drive as well as his production of sperm.

So, is there a "scent of fertility"? No one can say for sure. But, if you do love the way your partner smells – and he likely feels the same about you – spending time with each other when these 'natural' scents prevail might end up helping you get pregnant faster!

Allergy Drugs, Sex & Getting Pregnant

If you or your partner suffer with the sneezing, coughing, stuffy nose and watery, itchy eyes of seasonal or environmental allergies then one or both of you may already be using an allergy medication to control symptoms. And for most people they can offer life changing relief.

At the same time however, if you or your partner have noticed that your desire for sex is not quite what it used to be – or if you're having difficulty conceiving– then it's important to look to your allergy medicines as one possible source of problems. Indeed, studies show that in some folks certain allergy medications can have sexual side effects ranging all the way from a decrease in sexual desire in women, to complete inability to have an erection in men.

Moreover, while there is no direct proof, many doctors now believe that certain allergy medications designed to dry up mucous in the nasal passages, may also dry mucous in the vagina causing a number of problems from uncomfortable sex to difficulty getting pregnant. Indeed, as I previously explained, without the adequate lubrication provided by cervical mucus not only can intercourse be uncomfortable or even painful, a severe mucus deficiency can make it more difficult for your partner's sperm to swim through your reproductive system and reach your egg.

If you or your partner are taking allergy medications on a long term basis, and find that your sex drive appears to be decreasing, or if you notice that your vagina is dry and sex is more uncomfortable or your partner has problems obtaining or maintaining an erection, it's important that you speak to your doctor.

Tell him or her you are trying to get pregnant and ask if there is another prescription or over-the-counter allergy medication with fewer of these kinds of effects. If you must continue with your current allergy medications, ask if there is something you can add to your treatment regimen to counter the sexual side effects.

If your doctor agrees, you or your partner can try stopping your allergy medications for up to two weeks and see if your sex related symptoms disappear or get better. If they don't your problems may be rooted in other causes. Do, however, check with your doctor before changing or stopping any medications.

Sex Dos and Don'ts: More Ways to Increase Your Fertility

In addition to the positions that increase your chance of getting pregnant there are also a few sexual "Dos and Don'ts" that, for some couples could influence how quickly or easily they conceive.

By no means am I saying that the practices listed under "don't" are wrong or that they should not be enjoyed. But if you are trying to get pregnant, it's important to understand the impact of certain activities as they relate to getting pregnant quick and easy.

Oral Sex and Fertility

If you and your partner regularly practice oral sex it should have no adverse effects of any kind on your fertility. That said, you might want to hold off on this practice during the specific love making sessions during which you are actively trying to conceive. Why? Bacteria normally found in saliva can sometimes have a degrading effect on sperm, reducing their ability to fertilize an egg.

So if your saliva is present on your partner's penis just before he ejaculates or, more likely, if a large amount of his saliva is present in your vagina just prior to him ejaculating, problems could result. To increase your chances for getting pregnant either skip the oral sex while trying to make a baby, or clean off the saliva with a warm wet towel before having intercourse.

Anal Sex and Fertility

When done properly, with mutual consent, anal sex can be highly erotic and pleasurable for both partners. However, this activity does come with an important precaution: A man must wash his penis with hot water and soap between acts of anal and vaginal penetration. This must be the case whether you are trying to conceive or not, since bacteria which live harmlessly in the rectum can turn deadly if they enter the vagina. This can not only cause a whopper of a reproductive tract infection in you, should conception occur when this bacteria is present in your reproductive tract, any resulting conception may be negatively affected. The most common problem is early miscarriage.

Sex Toys and Getting Pregnant

I whole heartedly agree with the idea that getting pregnant should be fun! In fact, putting some honest-to-goodness playtime into your baby making efforts can actually help encourage your fertility. And, if sex toys, lubricants and other love making aids are a part of that "fun", that's okay - there are just a few guidelines to follow. While many of these items are safe to use during baby–making sex, here are a few precautions you should not ignore.

> *Vibrators -* Generally speaking a vibrator, in and of itself, is not going to harm your fertility. That said, like any object that goes into the vagina, it can harbor bacteria that can damage your reproductive organs and affect your ability to get pregnant. To make sure it doesn't, always wash your vibrator or other sex toy with soap and hot water before using - even if you washed it before you put it away. Taking this one step will help insure your fertility won't be affected.

> *Hot Tubs -* Though not technically a "sex aid" many couples find a relaxing soak in a hot tub a great prelude to sex – and it really can work! In terms of your fertility however, it may not be worth the price. First, the high temperatures of the water can cause some immediate harm, affecting not just your egg, but possibly your ability to ovulate. While the effect on sperm is not immediate, as you learned earlier, anything that raises the temeparture of the testicles by even a few degrees can harm sperm production.

While this won't affect the sperm he is *about* to ejaculate (it's made weeks in advance) if you are accustomed to soaking in a hot tub on a regular basis, eventually his sperm will be affected. So, while you are trying to get pregnant no hot tubs or very hot baths or hot showers right before having sex.

Lubricants: Many women find that using a lubricant can intensify sexual pleasure - and in this respect they may even subtly encourage fertility. However, your choice of lubricants is critical, since some can have a degrading effect on sperm – and some may even kill sperm on contact!

What to use: Water based lubricants or those suspended in a light gel formulation. Look for the words "Safe to Use with Condoms" on the package. If it won't break down the latex in a condom it's not likely to harm sperm.

What to avoid: Oil based lubricants such as petroleum jelly or massage oils, both of which can upset the natural acid balance inside your vagina, which in turn can destroy sperm. Moreover some oil-based lubricants can also slow sperm down, making it harder for them to swim and sometimes even block the passage to your egg. Just think of all the damage to marine life caused by oil spills, and you get an idea of how sperm react when smothered in the oil of a heavy lubricant!

Also be absolutely certain to avoid any lubricant containing non-noxyol 9. This is a spermicide developed to kill sperm and frequently used with condoms as a form of back-up birth control. Since many lubricants automatically contain this ingredient be sure to check the label!

Massage Oils: Like lubricants, massage oils can intensify your love making and help turn that "do it" time into a pleasurable sensual experience you both look forward to. While pretty much all massage oils are safe to use while trying to conceive, you should avoid using them in or around your vagina and your partner should avoid putting them directly on his penis. Using them anywhere else on the body – particularly the breasts, buttocks and legs - can be highly sensual and exciting. But for the moment, keep them out of direct contact with your genitals to be safe and sure.

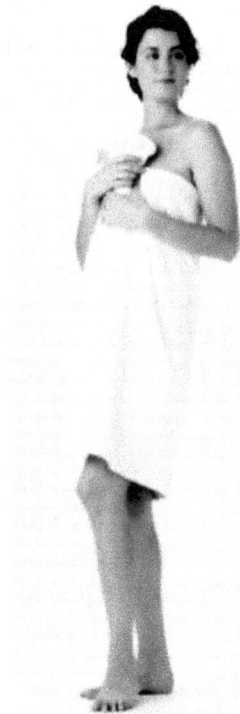

Q: *Is it true that douching can harm your fertility?*

A: While many patients report feeling "cleaner" after douching, this is not a practice I routinely recommend. The reason? First, your vagina is self-cleaning – meaning that normal regular secretions help keep the interior clean with a system of natural hygiene.

More importantly, there is good evidence to show that douching can dampen your fertility. How? Much like the skin on the outside of your body, the cells lining your vagina have a certain pH or acid balance. Normally, that should be between 4.5 and 5.0. – which, not coincidentally is also the acid balance that sperm just love.

Douching, however, changes that acid balance, causing your vagina to become either too acid or too alkaline – and either extreme can impact sperm motility and even survival. Unless your doctor diagnoses an abnormal vaginal pH – in which case a douche may be recommended to correct the problem – you should never use any douching product on your own.

In fact, you should not only avoid douching before intercourse, if you are trying to get pregnant, also avoid douching directly following intercourse. Why? Sometimes sperm can be a bit slow, lingering for a while in the upper portion of your vagina before heading to your uterus. Douching literally drenches and drowns those sperm – and ultimately this means fewer available for conception, thus reducing your momentary chance for conception. If your partner has even a marginally low sperm count, or if his sperm are poor swimmers, douching after intercourse can do enough damage to fully block conception.

And finally, you should also be aware that douching at any time increases your risk of a reproductive infection - one that may ultimately steal your fertility. How?

If there is an infection present in your vagina, or if there is any bacteria lingering on the outside of your vaginal "lips" (called the labia) douching can push those germs deeper into your reproductive tract, resulting in a much more serious pelvic inflammatory infection as well as increasing the risk of an ectopic pregnancy if you do conceive. This is a condition whereby a fertilized egg gets stuck inside the fallopian tube causing life threatening risks to the mother – so it's something you clearly want to avoid if you can.

If you do happen to smell an odor "down there" that doesn't seem right, often it can be the result of bacteria on the outside "lips" of your vagina, occasionally even from urine which comes in contact with this area. When this is the case, washing the outside of your "V" zone with soap and warm water will usually take care of the problem. If it doesn't, or if the odors persist and/or are extremely unpleasant, or if you develop an abnormal or odorous discharge following intercourse – or any time – then that may be a sign of a infection requiring antibiotics, so be sure to see your doctor.

Ultimately, if you find you must douche, a natural solution is best. To reduce vaginal acid try two tablespoons of baking soda in one quart of water; to increase vaginal acid try two tablespoons of vinegar in one court of water. Under no circumstances should you ever use a commercial douche labeled "unsafe for use during pregnancy." Any douche that is harmful during pregnancy should never be used when trying to conceive.

Sex and Conception: What's Age Got to Do with It?

If you pay attention to popular media, it's easy to come away with the message that a woman's sex drive peaks in her 20's – and then gradually declines, along with her desire to have a baby. But a new study published in the journal *Personality and Individual Differences* refutes the common media message with research that shows just the opposite! Indeed, according to the new research a woman's "baby making lust" actually continues well into her 40's – along with an *increased* desire for great sex that can go on indefinitely.

Indeed, researchers at the University of Texas at Austin found that women aged 27 to 45 actually have a heightened sex drive –and believe it's not just related to a ticking biological clock. Indeed, this study found that the more years that pass from the standard "peak" fertility time of the mid 20's, the more desire there is to have a baby – and it lasts right through to menopause - and sometimes even beyond.

To arrive at this conclusion, researchers compared responses to questions concerning sexual fantasies, frequency of thoughts about making love and a willingness to engage in casual sex or even one night stands from some 800 women divided into three groups. The groups represented "high fertility "(ages 18-26); low fertility (ages 17 to 45) and menopausal (age 46 and up). Researchers then analyzed the answers from each age group and compared them across the board.

The result: Surprising, even to the researchers, answers from the women in the "low fertility" group were remarkably similar to those in the "high fertility" group.   In short, at least according to this study, from late teens through the mid-forties, women had pretty much equal sex drives – and equal responses to the hormonal surges that drive "baby making lust." While the desire to have a baby after menopause obviously declined with the knowledge that it was no longer possible, still the desire for a warm, caring, intimate relationship was still on most women's minds.

According to psychologist Judith Easton, who lead the study group, while it may be more difficult, physiologically, to conceive after age 35, a woman's feelings about sex and her desire to procreate will "continue to motivate them to try until menopause."

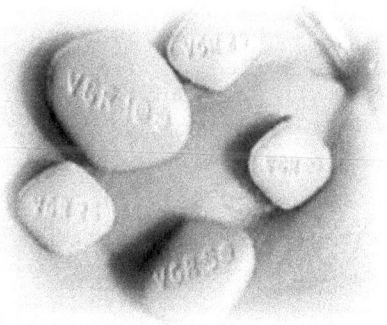

Q: *Is it safe for my husband to use Viagra while we are trying to conceive?*

A: Although the research into the effects of Viagra on fertility is still ongoing, some research has shown it can have a negative effect on sperm. In one study presented at the annual meeting of the British Fertility Society in 2004, researchers presented evidence showing that Viagra speeds up chemical changes within sperm that ultimately impact the enzymes necessary to allow penetration into the egg. Without those enzymes, the head of the sperm, called the acrosome, cannot penetrate the outer shell of the egg so fertilization becomes impossible.

More recently, studies published in the journal *Fertility and Sterility* in 2008 found that when treating sperm samples with the amount of Viagra normally found in the blood of a man after one dose, those sperm appeared more active – but again experienced damage to the acrosome. In a second study on mice, those given Viagra produced 40% fewer embryos than mice not given the drug.

Although there are no similar studies conducted on Levitra or Cialis, because their mechanisms are similar to that of Viagra, it is likely that they may result in similar effects on sperm.

That said, Pfizer, the drug company who manufactures Viagra sticks by their product, saying that use on tens of millions of men has not revealed any links to fertility problems.

You should also remember that because sperm is continually being manufactured, if your husband has successfully used Viagra in the past, simply abstaining from use for a couple of weeks prior to conception will ensure that no related problems will occur. Indeed, there is no evidence that any of the drugs used for erectile dysfunction can have lingering effects on fertility and they have in fact been credited for helping many couples enjoy a successful and happy sexual relationship.

As to non-prescription products, (particularly those sold over the Internet) which claim to increase male potency, there is little evidence that they work, let alone whether or not they impact fertility – so it's difficult to say one way or the other if they would be a viable substitute.

The bottom line: If your husband is having erection problems, he should definitely pay close attention to the diet and nutrition guidelines, as well as herbal treatments featured earlier in the book. In many instances I have seen men overcome impotency problems simply by changing their diet. If your partner smokes, suggest that he stop – this one step alone can dramatically alter his impotency issues. What can also help: Reducing alcohol intake, which can also have an impact on erectile dysfunction.

In addition, you may be able to provide some help as well, by removing some of the sex-on-demand stresses related to getting pregnant, and by making certain that your love making is as passionate and exciting for him as possible. Often, erectile dysfunction is a product of stress and helping your husband to relax and enjoy sex in a stress-free environment may be all he needs for a successful erection.

As to using drugs to combat erectile dysfunction: Turn to them only after you have tried the natural suggestions mentioned above. It's also important to note that if your husband's erectile issues continue you can successfully use the IVF procedure known as ICSI to help you conceive. In this instance your husband would give a sperm sample, which would then be placed directly inside your egg. Since there is no need for the sperm to drill through the egg's outer shell, drugs like Viagra should not have any effect on the conception.

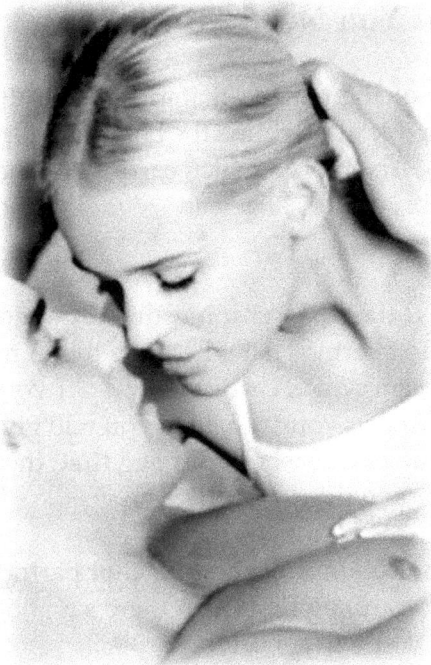

Sex & The Sex Of Your Baby

There is no question that virtually every couple trying to get pregnant would be equally happy to conceive a boy or a girl. This is particularly true if you've been struggling to get pregnant for quite some time.

Still, for some couples there remains an overwhelming desire to conceive either a boy or girl. This may be especially true if this is your second or third child, or perhaps the child of a second marriage.

Although there are clearly some proven high tech methods that many fertility clinics offer, there are also a few tried and true natural approaches that, at least anecdotally appear to work.

Of course simply by the rules of chance you are 50% likely to have a boy and 50% likely to have a girl – if it is your first pregnancy. So in this respect it's a bit harder to determine how well these natural sex selection methods work or how by how much they increase the odds that a specific gender will result.

That said, the more times you give birth to children of the same sex – for example 3 boys in a row – the more likely you are to have another boy during the fourth try. And in these instances I have seen couples use natural sex selection methods to change their gender pregnancy profile and finally have that little girl – or little boy – they wanted to make their family complete.

If you are interested in giving natural sex selection a try what follows are a few tips on what you can do. Remember, however, your goal should always be to have a healthy, happy baby and to love and cherish every child you conceive, regardless of their gender.

Choosing the Sex of Your Baby: What You Need To Know

Every child that is conceived is a combination of the genetic material inside the mother's egg and the father's sperm. The genes which determine the baby's gender are known as the "x" and the "y" chromosomes. An embryo which carries two "x" chromosomes will produce a girl, while an embryo that carries an "x" and a "y" chromosome will produce a boy.

Because a woman's egg always contributes the "x" chromosome, gender determination is always the responsibility of the sperm. That's because there are sperm which carry the "x" chromosome and sperm which carry the "y". If your partner's sperm carrying the "x" chromosome fertilizes your egg, then you will give birth to a girl. Likewise if it's his "y" chromosome that reaches your egg first, then it will combine with your "x" chromosome and you will give birth to a boy.

And this is really the key to what natural gender selection is all about: If your partner can get either his "x "or his "y" chromosome to your egg first, then there's a good chance you can influence the gender of the child you will conceive.

So, how do you do that? According to at least some scientific research, how you have sex holds the key!

Sex and Your Baby's Gender

The very first theory linking sex to a baby's gender was developed by Dr. Landrum Shettles. The basis of his theory is that sperm which carries the "x" chromosome (the one that makes a girl) swims slower but is heartier than sperm which carry the "y" chromosome (the one which makes a boy) which swim faster but have a shorter life span. Since we know that sperm can live inside a woman's reproductive tract for up to 5 days, Dr. Shettles theorized that manipulating the timing of when you have intercourse – and some specifics about the way you make love – could influence whether the "x" carrying hearty sperm or the "y" toting speedy sperm make it to your egg first.

So, if, for example you make love 4 to 5 days prior to ovulation, the slower moving but heartier "x" sperm are likely to be the ones to survive long enough to fertilize your egg when it finally ovulates. As such, you are more likely to conceive a girl. If, on the other hand you make love right at the point of ovulation, or just before, this favors the faster moving "y" toting sperm, which are responsible for creating a boy.

But there's a bit more to this theory than just the *great sperm race*. You can further influence which type gets there first via specific love-making techniques, with certain ways of being intimate more likely to encourage the success of either the "x" or the "y" sperm . Indeed, shallow penetration in the "missionary" position favors the slower moving "x" sperm, producing a girl, while deeper penetration during the knee-chest position favors the quick swimming "y" sperm, more likely to produce a boy.

Finally, there is some research to show that eating certain foods in the days just prior to attempting conception can also make a difference. The theory here is that gender is influenced, at least in part, by what scientists call the "ionic" factor. Simply put this is a type of biochemical "electric" charge that attracts sperm to egg.

The theory is that by eating certain foods which contain high levels of ionic- charged minerals - including calcium, magnesium, potassium and sodium - a egg can manipulate a kind of magnetic pull on either the "x" sperm or the "y" sperm. In research on 49 French couples conducted by a European physician named Dr. Joseph Stolkowski, 39 of the couples were able to influence the gender of their baby by manipulating their diet.

So with all this information in mind, here is your formula for natural gender selection:

> •**To Make A Baby Girl:** Have sex three to five days prior to ovulation and use shallow penetration performed in the "missionary" position. This allows your partner to deposit his sperm in the vagina, causing it to swim a little farther to reach the cervix. This in turn favors the slower-moving, more hearty female sperm, which live longer and will survive the journey better.

> •You should also try to avoid orgasm if you can. This will allow your vaginal environment to remain highly acidic, which helps to kill off the "y" sperm before they reach your fallopian tube.

• *To increase your chances further:* Eat foods high in calcium and magnesium such as milk, cheese, nuts, and beans and cereal.

- **To Make A Baby Boy:** Have sex as close to ovulation as possible – and if possible at the time of ovulation. Your partner should use deep penetration and the "rear entry "position which in turn allows sperm to be deposited at the entry to your cervix. This favors the faster moving male sperm, allowing them to reach your egg first, thus increasing your chances of conceiving a boy.

  In addition, this area of your V zone is generally more alkaline, thus favoring the survival of male sperm. If you also try to achieve orgasm at the same time you will help foster an even more alkaline environment and further increase the likelihood that a "y" male sperm will fertilize your egg.

  - *To increase your chances further:* Eat foods rich in potassium and sodium such as meat, fish, vegetables, chocolate and salty snacks.

While there are only a few small studies to show that these methods work, there are undoubtedly tens of thousands of anecdotal stories from couples who say that they do.

 In my own practice I have seen both methods work more times than would be allowed by chance. And following the publication of our best selling fertility book " *Getting Pregnant: What You Need To Know Now*" where I discuss these methods, along with other high tech scientific ways of doing gender selection, we heard from thousands of couples who used these simple methods and succeeded!

You should also be aware that there is a medical technique known as pre-implantation genetic diagnosis (PGD) which, when used for family balancing, can guarantee with 100% accuracy the gender of your baby. However, this does involve the use of in vitro fertilization (IVF) and it can be quite costly.

Either way, if you do decide to give gender selection a try, I want to once again remind you that first you should have fun, enjoy the sex and the baby making process and don't turn conception into a chore.

Perhaps even more important is to always remember that what matters most is conceiving and giving birth to a healthy, happy baby – regardless of their gender.

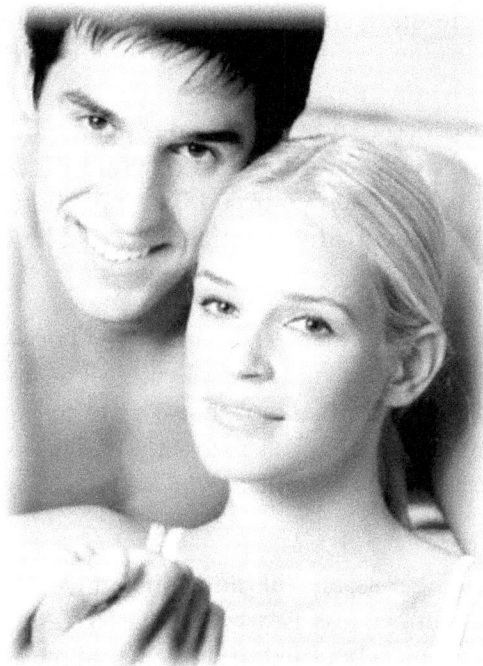

Some Final Advice:

How to Keep the Passion Alive

If you've been trying to get pregnant for even a few months – and especially if you've been trying for a while to no avail, you may be all too familiar with the term "sex on demand". And, in fact, if you are taking any fertility medications, you may even have been assigned a set of "Do It Now " days by your doctor - specific time frames that coordinate with your medications to produce the most likely chance for pregnancy to occur.

And in fact, even if you are trying on your own, using the ovulation prediction methods suggested in the previous chapter, you may also fall into the "sex on demand" mode, sometimes without even realizing you are doing so.

While it's true that having sex at the "right time" is your quickest route to conception, as you read earlier in this chapter, the "right time" doesn't just involve ovulation. It's also intimately tied to an entire network of hormonal activity, at least some of which is mediated by your sexual activity.

For your partner, sexual excitement affects more than the ability to have an erection - it also can influence sperm production, and in doing so can directly impact your ability to conceive.

So yes, it remains important that you do make love "at the right time". But it's equally important that you and your partner do not to turn this act into just another "chore" on your to-do list!   Indeed, it is extremely important, both from fertility and a psychological standpoint to keep not just the sexual embers burning, but the flames of desire as well.

But how exactly do you do that – particularly when the pressure to "get pregnant" at certain times of each month are high?   Here are some tips that many of my patients found helpful.

1. **Remember the love!** -The whole reason you and your partner decided to have a baby was because of your love for each other. And while it can sometimes be difficult to keep that in mind when your bed is full of charts and monitors and urine sticks, it's vital that you always remember that love is the reason you are having this baby.

2. **Keep the Romance Alive!** - There's love…and there's romance. And now, more than ever the two must meet!   Which is why I always suggest to my patients that they view their ovulation window as not just a time to get pregnant, but a time to make passionate love! To ensure that you do, approach the "do it " days the same way you would if you were getting ready for special "love" date.

    You can buy some scented candles, enticing massage oils and some new sexy lingerie while your partner might remember this is a great time to come home with a CD of your favorite love songs, a bouquet of flowers and a box of chocolates.   My point is to turn your "do it "days from a chore to help you get pregnant, into a sexy, romantic opportunity to spend some passionate time together. Remember, passion can lead to baby making sooner than just plain old sex!

3. **Make Time For Baby Talk -** I don't mean "pillow talk", I mean "baby talk" – as in discussions about your attempts to get pregnant. It's important that you and your partner continue to share your anxieties, your fears, and even your frustrations with each other – but NOT on the "Do It " days!

    Instead, set aside one day a week for "baby talk" – an hour when you can sit down with a cup of coffee or tea, relax, and talk about your baby making attempts. By having this time set aside to share your feelings, you'll not only bond closer together,   but also help keep the negative emotions and fears out of the bedroom when that ovulation window opens wide!

4. **Be Sensitive To Each Other's Feelings -** Each time you try to get pregnant - and it just doesn't happen - each of you can become sensitized to the experience and sometimes even scared to try, and fail, again. And it's important for each of you to recognize that fear in yourselves and   each other. But while

men and women feel the effects of repeated conception failure, in my experience it is men who often feel the sting the most. Each time you try – and don't succeed at getting pregnant, most men feel a little more inadequate and a more hesitant to try again.

And while he may normally be the "strong" one in the relationship, once conception enters the picture often the tables turn, and the female partner slips into the role of demanding drill sergeant – and often without realizing it, begins demanding sex at the "right time," in a less than sensitive way. If this sounds a little bit familiar then I urge you to turn those demands into *enticing* requests - filled with the kind of flirtations that will have him waiting with baited breath for the "right time" to arrive! Try a few sexy emails or texts as the "Do It" time approaches, or even tuck a handwritten note into his briefcase telling him you can't wait until " Friday" – or whatever your "Do It " day is!

Letting him know that you desire not just his sperm but *all of him* will not only help put some passion back into your baby making efforts, but in the process actually increase your chances for getting pregnant!

5.   **Pamper yourself!**   Everything from tracking ovulation and planning sex on demand, to using fertility drugs if that becomes necessary can take its toll on you. You may begin to feel frazzled, frustrated and extremely uptight, and even a little guilty as you sometimes wish this whole baby making thing would just be over already! What can help: Taking a little time out to pamper yourself. If you can afford it, this is the time to get a manicure and pedicure and if you can swing it, a professional massage and maybe a new hair cut. The more you feel "cared for" the less stress you will feel. If you're on a tight budget, then pamper yourself - make time for a spa-like bath or shower, have your partner give you a massage (and you return the favor the next night), or just spend time listening to your favorite music or reading a book.

The point is to direct your attentions away from the stress of getting pregnant and on to feeling relaxed and happy. Not only will this help you feel better , but the more relaxed you are, the more likely it is that you can partner can put the love back in your baby making efforts and in doing so create not just a new life, but some passionate memories to last a lifetime!

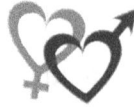

Chapter Eleven

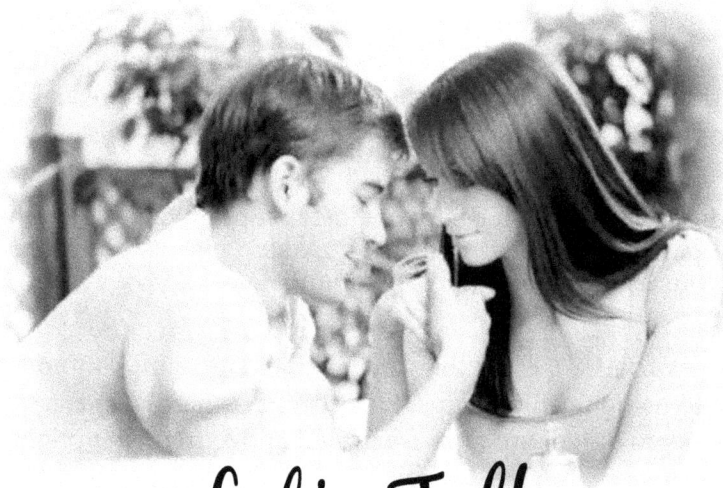

Let's Talk:
Conception & Conversation
The Power of "Pillow Talk "

Making the decision to have a baby – or to expand your family – could be one of the most important plans that you and your partner will make.

In fact, as a physician who has counseled and worked with thousands of fertility and obstetrical patients I can tell you that it is not just a decision that impacts each of *you* deeply, but one that also affects the precious new life you will bring into the world.

In addition to all of the obvious parenting-related responsibilities that accompany this decision, I cannot emphasize enough the unique bond that develops between a couple who bear children together. Indeed, having a child creates a connection between a man and a woman that can outlast even the most bitter and angry divorces. In fact even when couples come to the point where they despise one another, the bond they created as parents lives on in the eyes and the hearts of their children. For those who do remain together, that parenting bond becomes the "glue" that binds the family unit and creates a loving home in which children can flourish and grow.

But as important as this bond can be, sometimes the effort to create it can be somewhat of a bumpy ride. I am talking about the stress that can sometimes emerge during the process of getting pregnant. In fact, whether you have been trying for some time now to conceive, or have barely begun your journey towards parenthood, you probably already know that the anticipation of actually becoming pregnant creates frenzy like no other! As you look forward to each new month, and each new fresh attempt at conception, the anticipation builds and the excitement can be hard to contain. Most couples report that discovering they are indeed pregnant is one of the most joyous times in their life together.

But that said, I also know that things don't always seem to go as planned. Even when a couple is in seemingly perfect health, with no fertility problems, Mother Nature can sometimes take her own sweet time! For those of you who might already be experiencing some minor fertility problems, the time it takes to get pregnant could be even longer.

But the problem is not just the waiting. It's the variety of mixed emotions that become a part of that waiting game. I'm talking about the fear (that you won't get pregnant), the anxiety (that you may doing something wrong), the depression (when each month the anticipation of joy is met with failure) and even the failure itself, as you and your partner begin to worry that something serious might be wrong. If this is how you *are* feeling, please don't worry! These are normal emotions that, for most couples, are just a small bump in the road to becoming parents. As you turn to each other for comfort and support the time passes quickly and before you know it you are hearing that wonderful news that you about to become parents. And all of your fears and worries become a distant memory.

For some couples, however, the road to pregnancy isn't just a little bumpy - it's a treacherous climb up the side of a steep mountain in the pouring rain! As the fears and anxieties continue to mount with each passing cycle, these couples don't just *feel* first, with self-blame, and later turns to blaming each other. As this occurs, slowly but steadily a wall of frustration between them begins to build.

The most difficult part of this scenario: Very often it is the "wall" itself that becomes yet another obstacle to getting pregnant. How so? What many couples don't realize is just how powerful emotions can be, and just how powerfully they can impact many aspects of your physical health – including your fertility.

How Your Emotions Affect Conception

As I briefly mentioned in an earlier chapter, how partners relate to each other has the power to impact each individual's physical health - including affecting the brain chemistry involved in conception. And it can do so in either a positive or a negative way.

For example, studies have shown that when a woman falls in love and is in a happy relationship, her menstrual cycles become more regular and her ovulation pattern can go from abnormal to normal in just a matter of months! The same is true for men in the sense that being happy and content in a relationship can impact the brain chemistry involved in sperm production – and in this way help keep production humming along. And all of this can make getting pregnant a lot easier.

At the same time, however, women and men who are depressed, angry or otherwise unhappy with themselves or with their relationship often find themselves battling stress-related health issues that can turn their reproductive chemistry upside down. For these couples getting pregnant becomes more difficult - a situation that only tends to fuel their anger and depression more.

Of course this is not to suggest *in any way* that couples who have fertility problems are unhappy – or that they don't love each other. Most are truly loving, committed couples who work hard together, and almost always achieve their pregnancy hopes and dreams.

But what I'm talking about are those couples who are working so hard towards getting pregnant, that they focus only on that end goal – and in the process lose touch with the whole reason they are trying to get pregnant in the first place, which is their love for each other. As a result, the process of creating a baby can create a type of stress that not only makes it emotionally and mentally more difficult to "keep on trying", but can also lead to the kind of hormonal imbalances that can physically impact the ability to get pregnant.

Indeed, as you read earlier, stress and it's accompanying biochemistry, can take it's toll on fertility and become one of the be one of the most harmful aspects of modern living!

But for the moment I want to focus not on the chemical side of stress, but instead on the ways in which you and your partner relate to one another during stressful times - and how making small changes in the way you do that, can make a big difference in your ability to get pregnant.

Intimacy, Communication and Conception: What Every Couple Should Know

One of the most important relationship tools we have is conversation. When used in a positive constructive way, your words can literally change the world – or at least the world you and your partner share. But more importantly – at least from a relationship perspective
- the right words can also help you overcome many relationship obstacles, putting you and your partner on a path towards not just better understanding, but also a partnership that is deeper and more meaningful in all aspects.

At the same time, if we use our words without thinking – and in the process we hurt or belittle our partners – conversation doesn't just eat away at the bonds of intimacy, it also creates a cloud of negativity that can influence all aspects of our emotional and physical well being, including the ability to conceive.

So does this mean you have to keep your "gripes" to yourself – and never tell your partner how you are feeling? Absolutely not. It's important that we are as truthful with our partner as we are to ourselves. So, expressing your feelings, including your fears and frustrations – particularly about getting pregnant - remains an important part of the bonding process between a man and a woman, and more importantly between parents-to-be.

But it's also vital to remember the importance of *how y*ou voice your feelings, including the emotional tremor with which you express them,   that can make a huge difference in whether or not your comments will be the glue that bonds your relationship or the hammer that shatters it.

"Often couples express their own feelings of fear or anger by blaming the other person if their wishes of having a baby are not being fulfilled , says Danish relationship expert Poula Helth, who together with her partner Hans Jorn Filges have authored many best-selling books on the power of conversation, including the popular book , " Let's Talk". (See www.LetsTalk.info)

But, says, Helth, this does more than just point the finger of blame, it also turns a unified relationship into two separate units. " Instead of there being an "us" , there is now a " him " and a "her" - and over time this kind of thinking can sabotage anything you try to accomplish as a couple, including getting pregnant," says Helth. Equally as destructive, says Filges is when the fertility problems lead to anger and frustration that gets expressed in other ways – and in other situations.

"Couples trying to get pregnant often experience strong anger and lots of anxiety, but sometimes they try to ignore these feelings, "says Filges. As a result, he says that anger and frustration comes out in other ways, and in other situations involving the partner – but it can be just as destructive.

"It can show up as one partner being overly critical of the other in entirely different situations, even social situations, or it can come out as a desire to spend more time away from each other – or sometimes it is even expressed as kind of moodiness or depression – all behavior that seeks to "punish" the partner for anger related to the fertility issues," says Helth and Filges.

Equally - or perhaps even more destructive than anger which is *expressed inappropriately*, is anger that is *suppressed* – a situation that studies show may have a direct impact on the ability to get pregnant, over and above what the typical "stress response" might cause. According to research this may be particularly true for women who, by nature, are usually more vocal with their feelings. Indeed, for women who turn their angry feelings inward, getting pregnant could be more difficult.

In one double blind study published in the journal *Human Reproduction* researchers tested 156 infertile couples using several rating systems designed to determine levels of anxiety, depression and anger. They then compared the results to testing done on 80 couples who had no fertility problems.

The surprising result: While just being angry in and of itself had some impact on fertility for all couples, for those who were dealing with suppressed anger –

sometimes to the point of not even recognizing they were so angry - problems getting pregnant were significantly higher.

"The results do suggest the possibility of a subgroup of infertile couples have reactions beyond the distress that is consequent to the failure of repeated attempts to conceive a baby, these couples also have a poorly adaptive psychological functioning, which is likely to play an important role in the onset and course of functional infertility," says study author Dr. Secondo Fassino of the "Saint Anna" Hospital of Turin, Italy where the research was conducted.

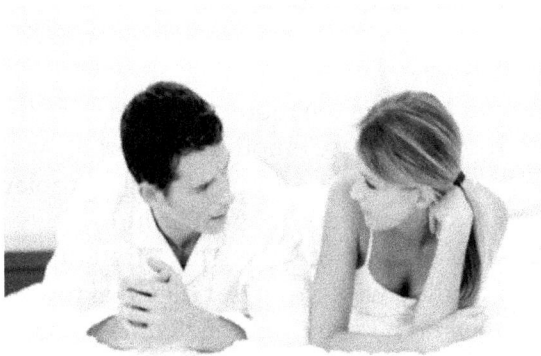

Dealing with the Anger: What to Do

So, if it's not a good idea to lash out at your partner – and an even worse idea to hold your anger in – you may be wondering what exactly is the answer!

The answer, is to deal with your anger in a way that is helpful to you without being harmful to your partner. How do you do that?

The first step comes in recognizing the angry feelings – and that isn't always easy to do. Of course it's easy to identify anger when you're treated rudely by a sales clerk or even when your mother-in-law "pushes your buttons"!

But when it comes to feelings about getting pregnant – or maybe not getting pregnant – angry feelings can sometimes be hard to define. Why? First, you *don't want* to feel angry – you want to feel hopeful, and you believe the two feelings can't co-exist. (They can and we'll get to how in just a moment).

Next, you may feel guilty about being angry – possibly because the anger is aimed towards your partner who you love. Or you may feel guilty because your anger is being fueled by the jealous feelings you may have towards other women, possibly even family members, who aren't having any problems getting pregnant.

Indeed, in one study published in the journal *Human Reproduction* a group of doctors from the International Health Foundation in The Netherlands reported that

"Why me?" was a common emotion expressed by many women having difficulties getting pregnant. That "Why me?" question, say the researchers, was often fueled by anger directed at everything - from the world at large, to friends and family, even anger at God.

But perhaps the form of anger that can be most destructive – and the hardest of all to recognize is anger that is directed inward, at ourselves. Indeed, self-anger is one of the most difficult emotions to bring to the surface. So difficult in fact, that many people deal with self anger by projecting their negative emotions on to others, blaming them for the discomfort they feel, rather than looking inside themselves for the source of their pain.

This can be particularly true for women who I believe are more stoic in nature than men. While women certainly are known for being more emotionally verbal, at the same time, they also frequently bear the brunt of problems (no matter the problem) believing they have to "carry the world on their shoulders" no matter how heavy or difficult things get. I believe that it is this very notion of "necessary strength" that keeps many women from recognizing and dealing with the anger they feel towards themselves. In fact some women believe they aren't even "entitled" to feel angry!

But the really important thing to remember is that first, you are entitled to feel angry, and no you don't have to feel guilty or fearful or ashamed that you do. The desire to have a child is one of our strongest, most profound biological urges – and when those urges aren't being fulfilled, anger is a natural feeling.

You also don't have to feel guilty about those jealous feelings you have when other family members or close friends are realizing their parenting dreams while you remain childless. It doesn't mean you don't want them to be happy – it's just difficult to share in that happiness when you can't seem to find your piece of the family pie. And that too is a completely natural way to feel.

Moreover, you should also remember that, as I said earlier, hope and anger *can* coexist, and recognizing any angry feelings you are harboring will in no way diminish your hopefulness about your future as a mother.

So, if you can have a heart-to-heart with yourself and explore some of your deepest feelings, and let them rise to the surface, I can promise you that the world won't stop turning and no one will think you are a bad person or a bad partner, or that you will

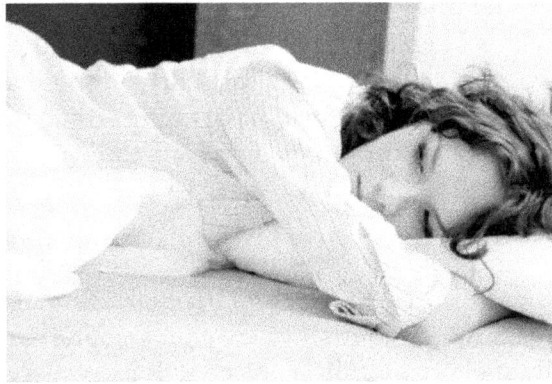

Angry? It's Really Okay ...

It's really okay to feel jealous or angry or upset when other family members or friends announce a pregnancy. You're entitled to feel angry! It doesn't mean you don't want them to be happy - it just means you want to be happy too!

And that's a perfectly normal emotion when trying to conceive.

be a bad mother! Quite the contrary, this will be an important step in going forward with your hopes and wishes.

Once you do recognize these feelings, I invite you to share them with your partner. Why? Throughout my many years of counseling infertile patients, I have learned that very often at least some of that self-anger results from a false belief that your partner is actually angry at you. And this, by the way, is true for both men and women.

Oftentimes we project our own feelings of inadequacy onto our partner, and believe they feel about us the way we feel about ourselves – and in doing so we can transfer some of the self–anger into partner-directed anger. As researcher Poula Helth pointed out earlier, this is a very common issue among infertile couples.

In fact, in one study published in the journal *Human Reproduction* by a group of Scandinavian researchers it was reported that women who had difficulty getting pregnant reported not just a higher level of negative emotional feelings, but that they also had a very negative sense of self-esteem. Some believed their partner no longer found them attractive (even though their physical appearance had not changed) and still more confessed to feelings of isolation, loneliness even a sense of grief , all feelings that grew each time another month of trying passed - and no pregnancy occurred.

But when you talk to your partner about these self – doubts (and guys, this is advice you need to hear as well), when you fess up about your feelings of insecurity and self–blame when a pregnancy does not occur as quickly as you thought it would, you might be very surprised to learn that your partner was feeling the exact same way about themselves!

At the same time, I also want to remind you of the importance of listening to what your partner has to say as well. And by this I don't mean just listen to the words he or she is speaking, but really "hear" what it is that is being said. If you are busy formulating your response – or trying to talk over what they have to say - then you might miss some of what is being said, and that can only complicate the negative feelings you may have about yourself and the relationship.

Most importantly I want you to understand that while putting all your emotional cards on the table is never easy, once you do, and once you and your partner begin sharing your feelings with each other, any anger or resentment that was building between you begins to almost magically melt away. In its place will be a deeper, more meaningful, far more intimate bonding fueled by the kind of communication that is not only healthier for each of you, but healthier for you both as a couple.

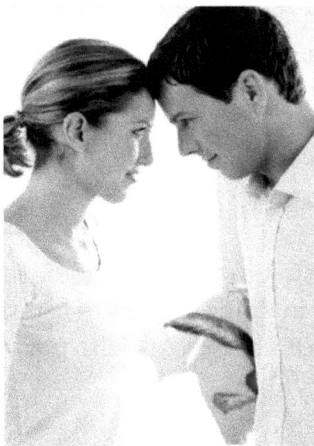

But what if it's really is the "other person's" fault?

Pointing the finger of blame never solved a problem – but it can create one where none exists. That said, if you suspect that your fertility problems could be related to something your partner is or isn't doing, it's important for you to bring it up – but do so in a gentle, non-accusatory way. In fact, if you are reading this book together – and I hope you are – now might be a good time to encourage each other to say all that is on your mind concerning your efforts to get pregnant.

Remind each other that you are a team, and that only when you work together as a team can any problems or stumbling blocks be overcome. And part of that teamwork: Discussing what each of you can do, on your own and especially together, to improve your chances for conception – and view every step you take as a team effort.

If "she" needs to change her diet, then "he" needs to support that by sharing in the same healthy meals. If "he" needs to stop smoking or drinking , "she" needs to support that by encouraging healthier behaviors and, when possible, make it easier for him to engage in healthy alternatives. What neither of you want to do is make demands or force each other to "do the right thing." Always remember: Getting pregnant is something you not only *need* to do together, but should *enjoy* doing together.

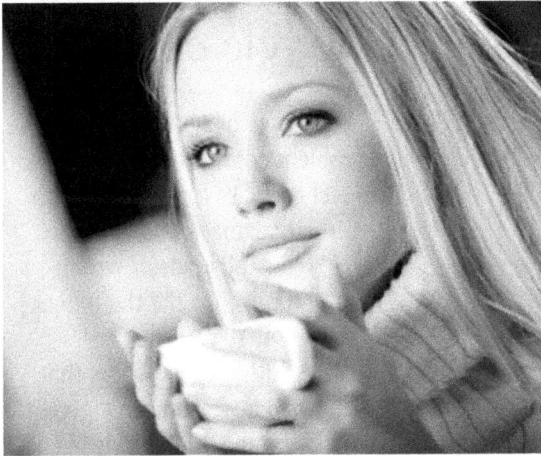

Just When You Think The Magic Is Gone...

Way back in 1999 – when fertility medicine was still considered a pretty new science – a group of Scandinavian researchers had the foresight to conduct a very telling study. In their research they measured the emotional tenor of couples from three different countries all trying to get pregnant. They then compared the findings to a group of couples who were not having any fertility problems.

Of all the interesting findings they ultimately published in the journal *Human Reproduction*, the one I found most significant pointed to the ways in which the emotions of infertility translated into behaviors that affected how couples related to each other in an intimate setting.

Indeed the vast majority of the couples who had problems conceiving reported that since trying to get pregnant their sex life, and their feelings of sexuality towards one another had declined – and for some quite dramatically. The frequency of love making among couples trying to get pregnant was ironically less than half of those *not trying*, while the rate of both sexual satisfaction and sexual pleasure was less than one-third of couples not trying to get pregnant.

On the surface this might look like fertility problems simply take the "magic " out of a relationship. But when you look just a little deeper, you find quite a different story. Indeed, from my experience treating thousands of couples, I have found that not only is the magic still there, if you and your partner make just a little bit of effort to really understand why you are feeling the way you are, not only can the sparks of romance return, but your fertility journey can become one of the most intimately bonding and sexually charged experiences you will ever have!

The key to making this happen: Recognizing that any concerns you may have regarding a lack of attractiveness to your partner, or any sense that you are unworthy of his love are just that - *feelings* – and not representative of the reality that is your relationship.

Getting Pregnant: Breaking The Cycle of Guilt

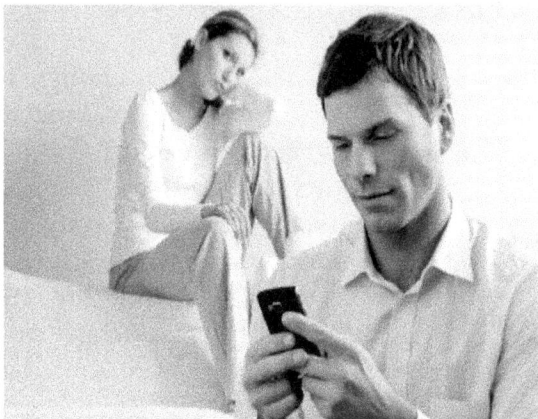

Many women who have a problem conceiving can begin to feel they are less attractive to their partner - and begin to "read" all kinds of wrong intentions into the the things they say or do.
The truth: Studies show that when a woman can't get pregnant most husbands blame themselves. Ultimately neither of you should blame yourselves or each other .

While you may feel that your inability to conceive makes you less attractive to your partner, I would bet that this is as far from the truth as one could get! In fact, you may be surprised to learn that when a wife cannot get pregnant, most husbands secretly blame themselves, and many harbor the same feelings of low esteem, and the feeling of not being wanted by their partner, as women do. So in this respect, it's entirely possible that your partner is feeling the same sense of unattractiveness and unworthiness about himself as you are feeling about yourself.

This is why I keep coming back to the very theme that fueled this chapter to begin with : The importance of sharing your feelings and working together, as a couple, towards your parenting dreams.

When each of you remains in touch with your own feelings, and are willing to share those feelings with each other – as well as listen with your heart to what your partner is saying - I promise that the journey to parenthood will not just take you down a happier and easier road, but quite possibly may be a more successful journey as well. Indeed, when you share your burdens they are always lighter to carry – and that in and of itself can free the body and the mind in ways that influence your health – and your fertility.

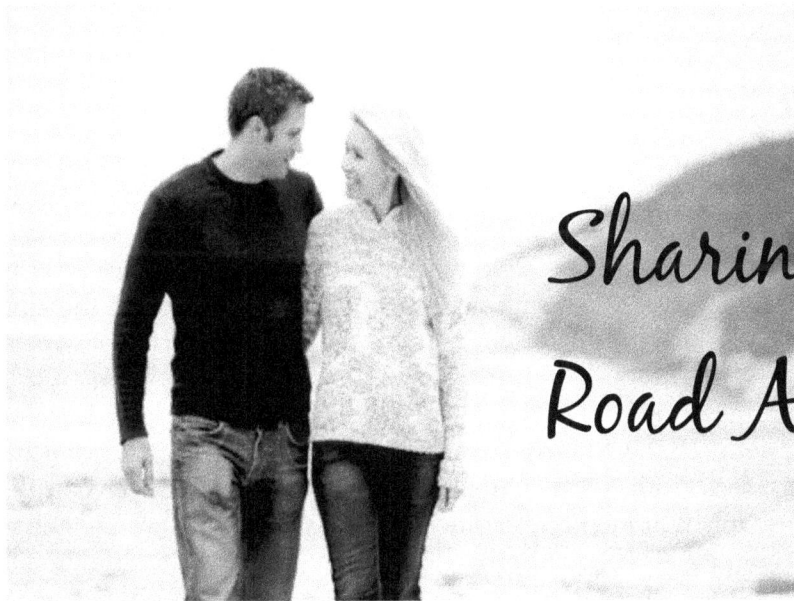

Sharing the
Road Ahead...

Some Final Words of Relationship Advice

Whether you have just started your journey towards parenthood, or you have been "on the road" for quite some time, your mind is no doubt filled with thoughts of ovulation prediction, sperm counts, eating the right foods, taking the right vitamins, making love at the "right time" - and most importantly, whether that little "little blue stick" is going to show you've succeeded at your goals.

And when you are trying to get pregnant it's perfectly natural to be thinking about all these things, as well as many other day-to-day thoughts and feelings related to having a baby. And, in fact, when it comes to the lifestyle factors that I've talked so much about in this book, it's important that doing what is good and right for your fertility remain foremost in your mind.

At the same time, I also caution not to allow your parenting goals to dominate your entire life – particularly to the point where you begin to forget the reason you wanted to have a baby in the first place, which is to celebrate the love and the bond you share. It is, after all, the love you have for each other, and the strength of your relationship, that helped you arrive at the decision to start a family – and these feelings for each other must always remain foremost in your mind.

Not only will this help carry you over any of the rough spots you might encounter on the road to parenthood, but even more importantly, working together, as a team, and keeping your feelings for each other in the forefront at all times, can also help your fertility to prosper!

Of course this is not to say that your relationship will be totally free of strife – no relationship ever is! There will be disagreements and even fights – and that is all totally normal. But if, throughout each day you remember not just the love you have for each other, but also the importance of communicating that love *to each other* in any way you can – well then the little disagreements and arguments will be the kind of healthy discourse that brings couples closer together, not drive them farther apart.

Perhaps most important, I urge the two of you to always keep the lines of communication open – which is a very important and easy way to keep little problems from building into big ones. Indeed one of the biggest mistakes I have seen couples make – and this is true for both men and women – is "assuming" they know how their partner feels about any given situation, without ever really taking the time to *find out* how they feel. And this can influence our behaviors in myriad ways.

Indeed, oftentimes when we "read" something into our partner's words or actions, we act on what we *think* we see - even when what we think we see might not be the truth. This in turn causes our partner to "read" something into our actions and then react in their own way. Before you know it, everyone is operating on assumptions and neither partner is communicating how they really feel.

So, how can you make certain that you don't "assume". Again, the answer is to always keep the lines of communication open – and to remember that communication is a two-way street. Not only is it important for each partner to express their feelings, it is equally important, in fact it is vital, that each of you also listen and really hear what the other has to say.

Indeed, Filges reminds us that it's not only important to listen to what your partner has to say, but also to repeat what they say, to be certain you understand what they mean, and internalize how they really feel.

"Listening and repeating is a core tool for improving communication – if you do just this one thing, you will see a vast improvement in the level of intimacy between you and your partner," says Filges.

When the lines of communication are kept open, when you ask instead of assuming, when you listen and really hear with your heart what each other has to say, the entire way that you and your partner relate to one another takes a leap forward.

Before closing this chapter I also want to relate to you a story about one of my patients. She and her partner had suffered a very long, and arduous struggle with infertility – trying to get pregnant for over 7 years , both on their own and with other doctors. And she told me that with each failure came another round of depression, anxiety, even fear, for both her and her husband. As more time passed, and each attempt at pregnancy failed, they began to fight and argue more and more - and even separated several times. When they came to see me, they said I was their "last hope."

That was a bit of an intimidating and tall order, but thankfully, I was able to finally find out what their fertility problem was. Together with the diet and lifestyle changes you're reading about in this book, she and her husband were finally able to conceive – and within not too long a time I delivered their bundle of joy – a healthy, robust, strong baby boy.

As I visited her in the hospital the next day, her husband by her side, I watched as they literally glowed with the unmistakable pride of new parents, holding each other and cooing over their beautiful new son.   The happiness and the sheer joy were literally palpable!   When her husband briefly left the room, I whispered to her " Now, aren't you glad you and your husband didn't split – and that you stuck it out? Wasn't it worth all the fights and arguments and bad feelings ?"

And that's when she spoke the words I will never forget. She looked up at me smiling broadly and winked as she said " Fights? Arguments? A split? I don't remember any of that – I just remember you helping us have a beautiful baby."

The point I am trying to make is this: Whatever negative feelings or problems that do arise during your journey to the blessed day, I can promise that when your own child is born, all of the negative experiences and emotions you may be feeling will melt away. In their place will be the sheer joy of not just knowing you have achieved your parenting dream, but that you have brought into the world a wonderful, beautiful new human being - a product of the love and the intimacy and the caring you and your partner share.

If you keep the possibility of this moment foremost in your mind, I can promise a safe, healthy and successful journey to parenthood.

And, if you and your partner can keep the lines of communication open and continue to talk - and to listen - no matter how difficult you think your problems may be, the two of you will find the right path and the right way to become parents.

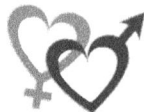

Chapter Twelve

Take Charge of Your Fertility

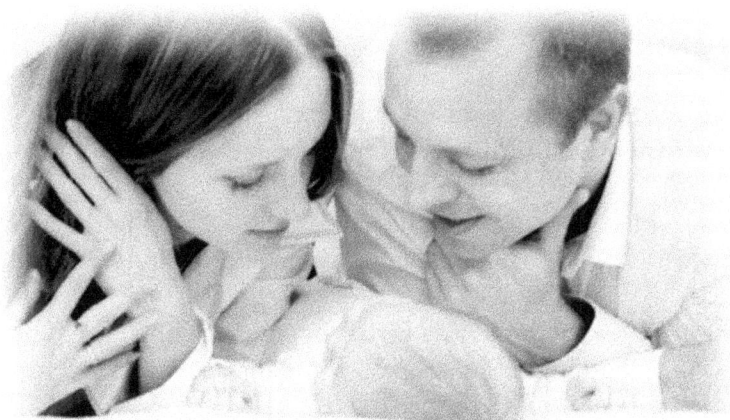

& Get Pregnant Fast!

It is my hope – and my expectation – that for most of you reading this book, making the small changes in your diet and lifestyle will be all it takes to get pregnant and have beautiful, healthy baby.

Indeed, throughout my many years as a fertility specialist I have helped thousands of couples just like you to get pregnant – even when they themselves had almost given up hope.

Which is why I also know that fear and anxiety has a way of taking over our hopes and dreams – particularly when it comes to becoming parents. It's not at all uncommon for couples trying to conceive to wonder or even worry "Can we have a baby?"

Adding to this natural sense of anxiety are the myriad articles, blogs and books about the epidemic of infertility, oftentimes affecting even young couples.   In fact, you might even have some friends who have needed fertility treatments in order to conceive

As a result you and your partner may be left worrying, "Will this happen to us?"

If this *is* what you are thinking, it's time to relax and stop worrying!   Again I will tell you that I am quite sure that if you and your partner work together and follow the advice in this book, you too will have your own little "miracle baby" before you know it!

Of course I would be remiss if I suggested that the advice in this book will be *all* it takes for *every* couple to get pregnant. The fact is, while the percentage is small, there are certainly some of you reading this book that may require some medical help getting pregnant.

In fact, I routinely suggest in all my books that if you are under age 35 and not pregnant after one year of trying, or over 35 and not pregnant within 6 months, then you should stop, take a pause, and think about whether or not a medical problem might be standing in the way – and definitely talk to your doctor about the possibility that something could be wrong.

At the same time, however, I don't want you to "panic" and jump to the conclusion that costly "fertility treatments" are your only option – because this just isn't true! Indeed, what many couples do not realize is that most of the time it is a small, or even a very common undiagnosed medical problem that is standing in the way of getting pregnant. Often, all the treatment that is required is a round of medication to restore your fertility and allow you to conceive.

In fact, I vividly recall one couple who sought my help as a fertility expert because, after several failed IVF attempts with other doctors (all their pregnancies ended in miscarriage) they were told their only hope was donor eggs. They came to see me for a "one last hope" opinion.

In looking over the medical charts from their previous treatments, something caught my eye right away – something very simple that seemed to be lacking in their medical history.   I asked the couple if either of them had ever been tested for infections in

If you don't get pregnant as soon as you thought you would it's easy to start believing that something serious is wrong.

But it's important that you don't jump to conclusions - and talk to your doctor first.

Often there's a small problem standing in the way, that's easy to fix!

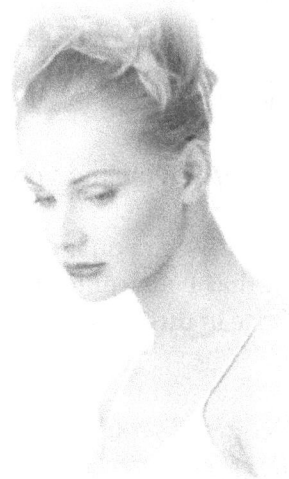

their reproductive tract – and they both answered "No".   This gave me a strong suspicion I knew I had to follow up on.

So, before planning any hormonal or other fertility tests, I ordered a sperm count with a complete culture for infection for him, and obtained urine and cervical cultures from her. My goal was to see if either one or both of them could be harboring an infection capable of causing their recurring miscarriages.

Sure enough, when the results came back both partners tested positive for E-coli – an extremely common bacteria that often causes no significant symptoms.   When present during conception however, this infection can be linked to both infertility as well as miscarriage – which of course was this couples problem.

I gave them both a prescription of antibiotics, and immediately put them on my vitamin regimen. I also gave them a diet featuring the foods similar to those suggested in this book.

Since they already had a vacation planned for later that month, I told them to make sure they took all the medication and then go ahead and enjoy themselves – and come see me when they returned.

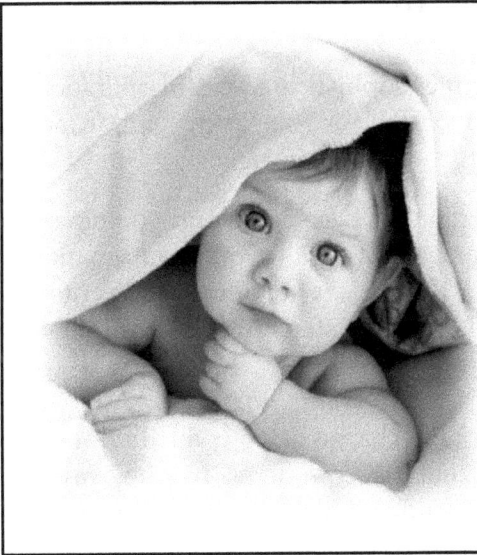

Even though fertility treatments make the headlines all the time, it's important to keep remembering that the vast majority of babies around the world are conceived naturally.

Sometimes, you just have to give Mother Nature a little bit of extra time!

A few weeks later they did return. They both said they took all their medication, but my patient said she wasn't feeling well. She indicated she was queasy, and had an upset stomach and was concerned because her period was late. She worried that her infection may have worsened.

I tried to reassure that everything was okay - but took a few tests to make certain – and asked her to phone my office in a couple of days. When she did I was overjoyed to give her the wonderful news: She and her husband were indeed pregnant! Some nine months later I delivered a beautiful baby girl – healthy as can be!

Not only did this couple get pregnant without the use of any fertility treatments, they also avoided another miscarriage, simply by curing the simple infection that I was certain had threatened each of their conceptions in the past.

I'm telling you this story because it so easily illustrates how sometimes a small, little problem – with a quick and easy fix - is all that stands in the way between you and pregnancy!

Take Charge of Your Fertility

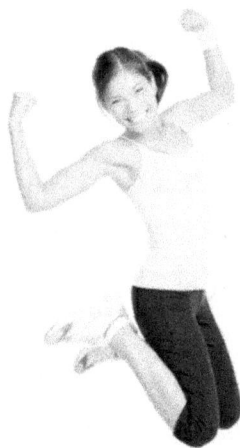

Certainly, for some couples sophisticated treatments such as artificial insemination or IVF are necessary in order to conceive - and they can be a true miracle!

At the same time, even if a year has passed and you have not been able to get pregnant, I don't want you to automatically jump to the conclusion that pricey fertility treatments are your only hope. There is, in fact, a step in-between, and I urge you to take it.

What is that step? To take charge of your fertility and see your doctor – advice that I recommend, by the way, for both you and your partner. Each of you should tell your doctor that you are having difficulty getting pregnant and discuss the possibility that something simple in your medical history – past or present – could be getting in the way. And, don't be afraid to bring up certain symptoms, and ask your doctor about specific tests and conditions that could be causing a problem.

How do you know what to look for and what to ask? That's where this chapter can help you. Indeed, in the pages that follow you will not only find the most common medical conditions to affect male and female fertility, but also the symptoms to look for, and the treatments that can help .

If any of these symptoms do seem familiar to you or your partner – and particularly if either of you have already been diagnosed with one of these problems – then I urge you to specifically bring these issues up during your doctor visit and openly discuss how they might be affecting your ability to conceive.

The bottom line: Always remember that there is hope, and there is help – and there is a very good chance that if you keep hope in your heart and take charge of getting the help you need, you and your partner will get pregnant and have the family of your dreams.

With this in mind, let's proceed to our last stop on our fertility journey – your doctor's office – where you may well the find the answers you are seeking.

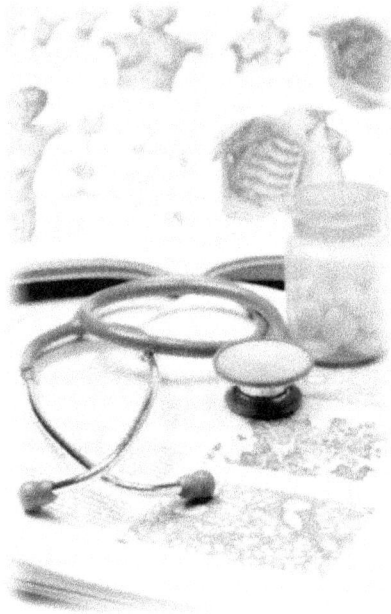

The 5 Most Common Medical Problems To Impact Female Fertility

Problem # 1: Endometriosis

Although most women plagued with this frequently painful menstrual disorder are aware that something is wrong, many don't know exactly what the problem is. Of those who do, a good deal are unaware of the close links between endometriosis and infertility – so close in fact that the American Society for Reproductive Medicine has cited this condition as the leading cause of infertility in young women.

If you're not yet familiar with this disorder, it occurs when tiny bits of uterine tissue meant to leave the body during a menstrual bleed, instead are pushed backwards through the fallopian tube into ultimately into the abdominal cavity.

Here, this misplaced tissue frequently lands on other organs and begins to grow. Endometrial lesions have been found on the ovaries, inside the fallopian tubes and in almost all organs inside the pelvic region. There have even been reports of endometrial tissue spreading as far away as the lungs.

The problem however is not just the tissue migration itself – because this occurs in 90% of all women, and most never develop endometriosis. What happens in those that do?

Normally, the moment this tissue migration starts, the immune system kicks into high gear, searching out and destroying the misplaced tissue before it gets a chance to actually land anywhere or begin growing.

But in the approximately 5 million women who do develop endometriosis their immune system fails them. Instead of recognizing this misplaced uterine tissue as abnormal, the immune system sees it as "normal".

So, it simply ignores the migration and the subsequent implantation that occurs. In fact, the faulty immune system sees the endometrial lesions as so normal, that it signals the body to begin producing a number of hormones designed to encourage growth. This, in turn, signals the tissue itself that it's okay to continue to spread and grow.

Because this tissue is hormonally charged (it's the same tissue that normally responds to hormonal stimulation inside your uterus) with each new monthly menstrual cycle, and each new round of hormonal stimulation, the misplaced tissue is joined by more bits of tissue, allowing it to become thicker and larger.

So, it's easy to understand how quickly and easily these deposits can build up and eventually, impact every organ within the pelvis.

It is, in fact, the growth and stretching of this tissue within the reproductive organs, along with the development of additional scar tissue that occurs over time that is responsible for the symptoms so characteristic of this condition. These include, chronic pelvic pain and discomfort that often worsens in the days before each period begins, and continues for a day or two afterwards.

Endometriosis: Know The Signs

How do you know if you have endometriosis? It's not always easy to tell, particularly since at least some of the symptoms overlap with other conditions, including simple menstrual cramps. But to help you better understand if this is your problem, here are some signs to look for:

· Severe menstrual cramps often starting on the first day of the period.
· Ovulation pain (Mittleschmerz)
· Pelvic pain that worsens just before a period begins.
· Painful intercourse
· Infertility/ Difficulty conceiving
· Recurring bladder infections
· Pelvic cysts and tumors
· Lower back pain
· Nausea, vomiting and dizziness during each period

Important to note: Although most women who are eventually diagnosed with endometriosis usually have at least two of these symptoms, sometimes they can also be signs of other disorders, including ovarian cysts, pelvic infections, or an ectopic pregnancy. This is one important reason why you should always have your symptoms diagnosed by a gynecologist.

Equally important to note is that for reasons we really don't understand, in some women endometriosis produces no symptoms at all. Moreover, some women who have almost every symptom on the list may have very little disease, while others may have extensive endometrial deposits in every area of their pelvis and feel no outward symptoms.   In fact, sometimes the first clue that something is wrong is that they are not able to get pregnant!

Adding to the mystery of this disease, in a study published by the American College of Obstetricians and Gynecologists in the August 2011 edition of the journal *Obstetrics and Gynecology* doctors found that the location of the endometrial lesions themselves, do not necessarily correlate to location of the pain – meaning, lesions could be growing in one area of your pelvic cavity while you feel pain in an entirely different area.

This is one reason why diagnosis can't be made via a physical exam only and why testing via imaging or even visual surgical diagnosis may be necessary.

How Endometriosis Affects Fertility

When it comes to getting pregnant, endometriosis clearly presents some challenges.

- When the renegade tissue lands on your ovaries it can interfere with proper egg develop and ovulation.

- When it sticks inside in your fallopian tubes, or on the fimbria at the ends of the tubes, it can cause scar tissue which in turn creates a barrier that can keep sperm from reaching your egg, or stop your fertilized egg from reaching your uterus.

- If endometrial tissue invades the wall of your uterus (causing a condition known as adenomyosis) it can cause damage that creates a hostile environment that can increase the risk of miscarriage.

In addition to all these problems endometrial lesions also emit hormone-like substances known as "prostaglandins" which can cause contractions anywhere within your reproductive system. When these contractions are strong enough they can push a newly fertilized egg down your fallopian tube too quickly, resulting in miscarriage.

Endometriosis: Hope and Help

As devastating as this disease can be, it's important to remember that most fertility problems occur only when this conditions remains undiagnosed and untreated. Once you do receive proper care – and the earlier the better – your odds of getting pregnant rise dramatically.

Most often endometriosis can be treated with a number of different medications, or when necessary a simple surgery to remove some of the misplaced tissue and free –up any organs that were affected.   You can read more about all your treatment options in my book *"Getting Pregnant: What You Need to Know Now."*

Moreover, you should bring your symptoms – including any problems getting pregnant – to the attention of your gynecologist, who is the best one to help begin your treatment regimen.

The really good news is that all of the recommendations in *Eat, Love, and Get Pregnant* – including the diet, nutrition and exercise suggestions –will be extremely helpful to reduce symptoms of endometriosis, so please continue to stay the course. In fact, for some of you, simple diet and lifestyle changes will be all that's necessary to take control of your endometriosis and get pregnant naturally.

Problem # 2: Thyroid Disorder

If you press your fingers gently to the base of your throat, you will find a small, butterfly shaped gland known as your thyroid. Normally it is so small you can't readily see or feel it. But as tiny and as delicate as this gland may it plays a huge role in not just your fertility, but also your overall health.

That role begins not in the thyroid itself, but in your pituitary gland, located in your brain. It secretes a hormone known as TSH – thyroid stimulating hormone – which in turn signals your thyroid gland to produce two key hormones of its own. They

Testing For Thyroid Disorder

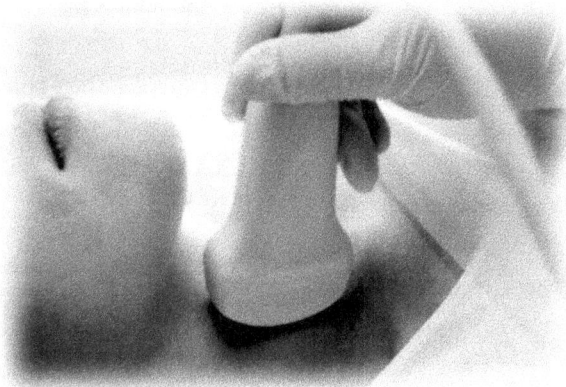

Usually a simple blood test checking for thyroid hormone will reveal if there's a problem. When more tests are needed, a painless ultra-sound exam of the gland itself could reveal the reason behind your fertility problems!

are thyroxine (T3) and triodothyronine (T4) and together they work to direct many metabolic functions, including those involved in the production of certain reproductive hormones.

When you are healthy and all of your hormones are in sync, your thyroid hums along at a quiet but steady pace, influencing your metabolism and your fertility in a positive way.

And, in fact, in an earlier chapter you read about the important links between your thyroid gland, your metabolism and weight gain – and how exercise can help keep all three running normally. And certainly, for many women, this is the ticket to increased fertility.

For some of you however, it might take a bit more than just regular exercise to keep your thyroid gland in good working order.   This is frequently the case should an undiagnosed immune system disorder cause your thyroid gland to veer off course.

When it does it can begin either overproducing thyroid hormone (a condition known as hyperthyroidism) or under-producing (a condition known as hypothyroidism) either of which can lead to any number of health problems, including infertility.

But how and why does this happen in the first place?   In the two most common causes of thyroid disorder – Graves Disease (hyperthyroidism) and Hashimoto's Throidytis (hypothyroidism), the immune system appears to be at fault.

- In **Graves Disease,** a malfunction in the immune system causes the production of abnormal antibodies that mimic TSH. This in turn sends a false signal to the thyroid gland that more thyroid hormone is needed – so it begins overproducing.
- In **Hashimoto's Thyroidytis,** an inflammation within the thyroid gland itself develops causing the immune system to believe a "foreign invader" has entered the body. In an effort to remove it, the immune system begins churning out killer cells destined to hunt down the invader and destroy it. But instead, it attacks the thyroid gland itself, causing a slowdown in the production of thyroid hormone. If left untreated that production may completely stop.

Other common causes of thyroid problems can include a nodule on the gland itself (called a goiter) which can influence the production of thyroid hormone, or an inflammation of the thyroid gland which is temporary, but can cause a malfunction in thyroid hormones.

How Your Thyroid Impacts Your Fertility

Because your thyroid hormones are so intimately entwined with the production of your reproductive hormones, it's no surprise that a malfunction can lead to problems getting pregnant.

- If your thyroid is under active you can experience an increase in the prolactin, (condition called "hyperprolactinemia") a hormone which is normally secreted only after you give birth. It acts like a form of birth control making it harder to conceive. So, when your thyroid causes prolactin levels to rise abnormally , it's as if you are using birth control - so getting pregnant is difficult.
- Luteal Phase Defect - In this condition you do not manufacture enough progesterone in the second half of your cycle - so even if you do conceive, your risk of miscarriage is abnormally high.
- If your thyroid is overactive you are likely to develop cysts on your ovaries that can interfere with or even prevent ovulation from occurring.

If you do get pregnant when your thyroid is out of sync some studies suggest it may increase your baby's risk of birth defects, including mental retardation. There is also an increased risk of miscarriage as well as an increased risk of fetal death in women with undiagnosed hypothyroidism.

What makes a thyroid disorder so tricky is that symptoms can be hard to pin down in both men and women. While there are some definite signs (see below) oftentimes symptoms can be subtle and hard to recognize–or can be confused with those of stress, anxiety or even fatigue.

Despite the absence of ovulation in women with thyroid disorder, your period may appear perfectly normal. So again, you might not even know your fertility is affected until you try to get pregnant, and have a difficult time doing so.

Thyroid Disorder: The Symptoms

Check with your doctor if you have at least two of the following symptoms from either list below.

Under active Thyroid:
- A ball-like swelling in the neck (called a goiter)
- Neck or jaw pain
- Sub normal body temperature
- Weight gain, thinning or coarse hair, and puffy face.
- Low energy
- Problems getting pregnant or recurrent miscarriage

Overactive Thyroid:
- Nervousness, anxiety, palpitations, shortness of breath
- Heat intolerance
- Fatigue
- Dry or gritty eyes, lid swelling, vision problems
- Constant hunger
- Diarrhea
- Sweating, leg swelling, hair loss, itchy skin
- Muscle weakness
- Irregular menstrual cycle, infertility; chronic pregnancy loss.

Thyroid Disease and Getting Pregnant: Yes You Can Conceive!

If you are diagnosed with a thyroid disorder, treatment is usually fast, painless and easy. In most instances a simple blood test for levels of T3 and T4 will help reveal if your thyroid is functioning normally. On occasion you may also need a scan to check for subtle problems within the gland. When an abnormality is found, medications are used to either help stimulate more thyroid hormone production, or, if necessary, slow it down. Once your thyroid hormones are normalized (it should only take a few months) your fertility will be restored, you will likely find that pregnancy comes quick and easy!

While far more women than men are affected by a thyroid disorder, it can happen to men as well. When it does occur, both sperm production and motility can be affected. Signs are similar to women (see Thyroid Disorder: Symptoms on the previous page). Once function is restored via medication, sperm production usually returns to normal.

Problem # 3: Poly Cystic Ovary Syndrome

For an increasing number of women, difficulties in getting pregnant can be traced to a condition known as PCOS – short for poly cystic ovary syndrome. Although it affects the ovaries – causing them to overproduce follicles but preventing them from developing into eggs - the underlying cause of this condition is blood sugar related. More specifically PCOS is thought to be linked to a condition known as insulin resistance. What is this - and how does it affect fertility?

Normally, insulin is the hormone that helps carry sugar from your bloodstream into your cells, where it is used for energy. When insulin resistance occurs your cells don't respond to this process in the normal way – and they don't let the sugars in. Your body then reacts by producing greater amounts of insulin – in hopes of getting the cells to respond. And it is at this point that the link to fertility problems begins.

Although doctors aren't certain as to why, the excess insulin in your bloodstream appears to send a signal to your ovaries to step up production of the male hormone testosterone. Normally produced by the ovaries in very tiny amounts, the increase in insulin dramatically changes that production level.

As testosterone levels rise it prevents any egg follicles that have formed from developing into an actual egg that can be ovulated and eventually fertilized. This in

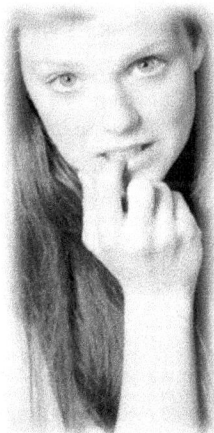

Could you have PCOS? Check for these symptoms:

- Highly irregular periods or no periods

- Abnormal hair grown on face and body

- High Blood Pressure

- Unusual weight gain even with dieting and exercise.

- Months without a period, followed by heavy bleeding for days.

- Elevated testosterone, prolactin and DHEA

- Abnormal ratio of LH to FSH

turn sets off an entire chain reaction of hormonal and other biochemical events that eventually come together to create the all of the symptoms of PCOS - and cause infertility.

PCOS: You Can Get Pregnant!

Although the symptoms of PCOS may seem obvious – and for some women they are – it's important to know that for many of you they can be so subtle they are barely noticed. In fact, for the majority of women who have mild PCOS the first sign that something is wrong is that they can't get pregnant.

So if you are having problems conceiving - and particularly if you have one or more of the symptoms of PCOS - talk to your doctor. If, in fact, you are diagnosed with this condition – or with insulin resistance – usually medications can help.

Among the most useful is the prescription drug Metformin – which helps increase the body's responsiveness to insulin, so that more does not need to be produced. When the egg-stimulating drug Clomid is added into the mix, this can completely turn PCOS around and dramatically increase your fertility. I'm happy to report that most women with PCOS who use this regimen can successfully get pregnant – and you might even have twins, which is more common among women with PCOS who do conceive.

But in addition to these medical treatments, there is also much you can do on your own to help reduce the fertility related consequences of PCOS and in the process also help overcome many of the symptoms of this condition. Among the most important are changes in diet and nutrition. By simply reducing your intake of simple carbohydrates – foods such as bread, pasta, cake and candy, plus starches like white potatoes and white rice - you can reduce your body's need for insulin, which in turn will help lighten the impact on your cells and your ovaries.

Adding more fiber to your diet can also help, along with foods high in omega 3 fatty acids – such as fresh fish. As you read in an earlier chapter, this nutrient can play a critical role in maximizing fertility in all women – and the effects are doubly good in women with PCOS.

For more complete information on the foods, nutrients and supplements that can have a major impact on PCOS – and increase your fertility at the same time – my latest book *Green Fertility: Natures Secrets for Making Babies* can be very helpful. Here you will find an entire section devoted to PCOS and the natural treatments that can help.

Most important, of course, is to get the proper diagnosis of your symptoms – and to begin treatment as soon as possible. If your gynecologist cannot help you, then you should seek the expertise of an endocrinologist, which is a doctor who specializes in blood sugar and related problems.

Problem # 4: Infections

If I had to pick the single most overlooked cause of infertility in both men and women, I would have to say infections would top the list. This is particularly true of sexually transmitted diseases (STDs) – including infections such as chlamydia, gonorrhea, herpes, HPV, and syphilis. In many instances the infection itself can be "silent" causing no symptoms for many years - making it even harder to recognize as a cause of infertility.

But it's not just infections with STDs that can temporarily get in the way of getting pregnant. Yeast infections, urinary tract infections and vaginal infections (particularly e-coli, which was the case with the patient I told you about earlier), or any infection within the reproductive system can interfere with the functioning of your reproductive organs and in doing so impact your ability to get pregnant.

If the infection is severe enough, a condition known as PID or pelvic inflammatory disease can result. Although this presents a dangerous and long lasting threat to your fertility, because it often carries a number of symptoms that are hard to ignore

The Signs of Infection: What to Look For

While many reproductive infections have few or no symptoms you can easily recognize, there are some that do. Although sometimes the symptoms are slight, and can be easily overlooked, if you remain vigilant about your V zone health, you can spot these signs and bring them to your doctor's attention.

Here's what you should look for:

·   Any usual discharge – including changes in color, texture or amount.

·   Any usual odors – no matter how slight. This is also true of odors that appear in relation to your menstrual cycle occurring either right before or right after your period.

·   A yellow or green tinged discharge.

·   A white clumpy or thick discharge

·   Any burning or pain, particularly after urinating.

·   Vaginal discoloration, such as redness, or any change in color.

·   Any V zone itching.

·   Firm, dark pink or red growths in or around your vagina.

·   Clear, fluid-filled blisters that itch, burn or hurt

– including severe pelvic pain and discharge – most PID infections are diagnosed and treated early, so they usually leave few or no lasting effects on fertility.

However, what concerns me and many fertility specialists are organisms like Chlamydia – which while they often cause few or no symptoms, can silently damage your entire reproductive system, causing a form of PID that virtually has no symptoms, but at the same time can leave you infertile.

In addition Chlamydia can also create what is called a "hostile environment" within your reproductive tract, particularly in your vagina, your fallopian tubes and your uterus. And by "hostile" I mean that the organism creates a condition that can make it difficult for egg and sperm to connect as well as compromising the overall health of both egg and sperm, making it difficult for either one to survive long enough for fertilization to occur.

Moreover if you do happen to beat the odds and get pregnant anyway, these organisms can make it difficult for your embryo to survive – as was the case with the couple who had undiagnosed E-coli infection that I mentioned earlier.

Treatment Can Restore Fertility Almost Immediately!

The good news is that once diagnosed and treated – usually with a course of antibiotics or other medications - the infection clears and there are often no lasting fertility effects. In fact, most couples usually get pregnant within a couple of months of treatment.

What's important to note, however, is that sometimes, when left untreated for a significant amount of time, some of these infections can cause permanent damage, often within the fallopian tubes. This is most prevalent with sexually transmitted diseases such as Chlamydia or gonorrhea, but it can happen with almost any bacteria or organism that remains in your body for a long enough period of time.

As such, if you are diagnosed and treated for one of these infections, and you are not able to get pregnant within a few months after, then it's important that you see a fertility specialist and have an x-ray of your fallopian tubes (called a hysterosalpingogram) to ensure that no damage was done. If damage has occurred, then there are additional treatments that may help – or you could be a candidate for one of the new "Green" natural IVF procedures, which you can learn more about in at www.GreenFertility.com

Problem # 5: Gluten Allergy

In the not too distant past, Elizabeth Hasselbeck, co-host of popular ABC show 'The View' gave birth to one of the most amazing and important public awareness campaigns ever, all about a very little known cause of infertility. That cause is a gluten allergy - also known as Celiac disease – a problem that affects millions of people, mostly women, worldwide.

Ms. Hasselbeck, herself, struggled with infertility for a number of years until she was diagnosed with Celiac disease – a diagnosis that changed not just her health but her life. Now the proud mother of three beautiful children and a continuing health force for other women and men caught in the web of misdiagnosis and maltreatment, Hasselbeck helped raise awareness about gluten sensitivity and its role in infertility, in a way that I believe had a powerful impact on many struggling to conceive.

Still, with all she has done, day after day, I talk to women who never stop to consider this problem as a reason behind their own difficulties conceiving - or as a factor in recurring miscarriage.

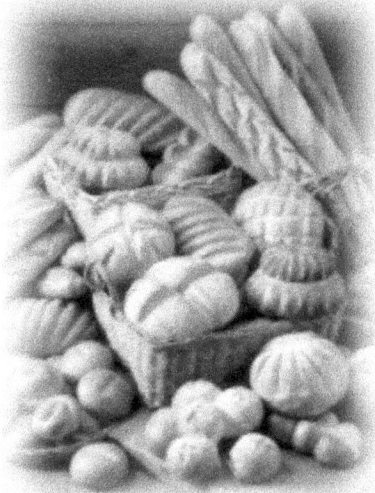

Can Bread Cause Infertility?

It's long been known as the "staple" of life. But for those who have Celiac disease - a condition that keeps them from properly digest wheat, any product containing gluten, a type of protein found in wheat, as well as rye and barley triggers an immune system reaction that causes the body to produce toxins.

In some women, this reaction also leads to certain types of infertility - including increased risk of chronic miscarriage.

For this reason I want to take a few moments to pass on some information that, while it may not help all of you, can certainly help those of you who are affected by this condition.

What is Celiac disease - And How Does It Affect Fertility?

In order to absorb nutrients from food, your intestines come equipped with tiny hair-like projections called villi. Think of these as tiny pond-fronds moving back and forth within your intestines, helping to pull the nutrients from foods and send them into your blood stream.

In those who have Celiac disease, eating products rich in gluten (a type of protein commonly found in rye, wheat and barley) ignites an immunologic firestorm that causes the body to produce toxins. It is these toxins that damage the villi. So, instead of standing up and pulling nutrients from food, they lie flat.

When this happens nutrients in the foods you eat are not properly absorbed - including those from proteins, carbohydrates and fats, as well as vitamins and minerals and in some cases even water and bile salts.

But if you're thinking it's just a lack of nutrients that leads to fertility problems, you're only partly correct. Because increasingly research suggests these same toxins create body-wide inflammation capable of affecting not just your digestive health, but your overall health – including your fertility.

In fact in one study, a group of Italian researchers concluded that Celiac disease – or gluten allergy – can be a leading factor in "unexplained infertility". Other researchers have linked it to recurring pregnancy loss and a higher rate of infertility overall.

But how, exactly does this condition keep you from getting pregnant? Celiac expert Dr. Alex Shikhman believes it may be through the increased production of the hormone known as prolactin – which, as you read earlier, acts like a natural barrier to conception.

"Studies show that when women allergic to gluten eat this protein, it typically causes an upswing in the production of prolactin," says Shikhman, director of the Institute for Specialized Medicine in Del Mar, California.

Produced by the pituitary gland, and normally secreted in small amounts in both men and women, prolactin is the hormone that naturally increases during pregnancy to help prepare your body for breastfeeding. But it also does something else: In high amounts prolactin turns *off* the production of FSH and LH, the chemicals linked to both egg production and release. In fact, one of the reasons most women don't get pregnant while they are breastfeeding is because high levels of prolactin keep them from ovulating.

At the same time, however, if you want to get pregnant, the production of FSH and LH is critical – so, keeping prolactin levels low is essential. When a gluten allergy is left untreated, keeping prolactin levels under control is near impossible. And so is getting pregnant.

Moreover, since the very nature of a gluten allergy means that you are absorbing far less nutrients from your foods and even your vitamin supplements that what is necessary for good health, I also believe this condition can lead to a deficiency of key nutritional factors essential to getting pregnant - particularly the B vitamins, plus vitamins C, D and A, as well as minerals like calcium and iron.

Gluten Allergy and Recurring Miscarriage

In addition to making it harder to get pregnant, if you do happen to conceive, a gluten allergy can also increase your risk of miscarriage. This occurs when related chemicals known as antiphospholipid antibodies cause the formation of tiny clots within your placenta, the sac that surrounds and nourishes your baby in the womb. Because these clots can block essential nutrients from reaching your baby, they may not receive the nourishment necessary to sustain life. As a result, the pregnancy spontaneously ends in miscarriage.

Moreover, when a mother has poor nutrition, before and right after conception, studies show that the risk of miscarriage also increases. Again, it stands to reason that if you are not absorbing the proper amount of nutrients from your foods or your prenatal vitamins, then your baby will not be receiving the proper nourishment necessary to survive and thrive. So even without the antiphospholipid antibody syndrome related to a gluten allergy, still, your risk of miscarriage would naturally increase if you have this condition.

The Good News: Get Diagnosed and Get Pregnant!

As Elizabeth Hasselbeck has so beautifully demonstrated, even the most severe forms of gluten sensitivity respond incredibly well to dietary changes – and in doing so, fertility is usually fully restored! These changes include eliminating all forms of gluten from your diet – such as grains like wheat - and replacing them with non-gluten substitutes, grains such as corn, oats or rice. Depending on how severe your sensitivity is, once you make the switch, healing can take anywhere from 6 months to two years – but in the process there is lots of improvement. For many women whose fertility was affected by gluten sensitivity, conception is often possible after as little as 6 months on a gluten-free diet.

To discover if you have a gluten allergy, talk to your doctor about the following blood tests:
- Anti-gliadin antibodies (AGA) both IgA and IgG
- Anti-endomysial antibodies (EMA) - IgA
- Anti-tissue transglutaminase antibodies (tTG) - IgA
- Total IgA level.

Remember, however, you must be eating gluten foods at the time of the testing, in order for the diagnosis to be accurate. So, if you plan on having these tests, don't change your diet until after they are completed.

To learn more about the impact of gluten sensitivity on fertility, plus get some helpful tips on changing your diet, and finding the "hidden" sources of gluten in the foods you eat every day, I recommend you read *"Green Fertility: Nature's Secrets for Making Babies"*.

The Medical Problems That Affect Male Fertility

If your partner is like most men, I guarantee he views his fertility as pretty much indestructible! In fact most men sort of assign "superman" status to sperm, believing there is little that can get in the way of their baby making ability.

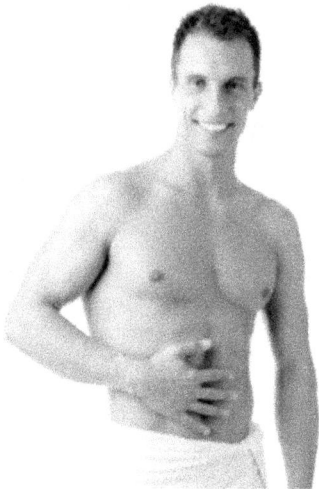

But the truth is, male fertility can be even more vulnerable than female fertility. In fact, up to 50% of all fertility problems are sperm related. Indeed, every time your partner gets a case of the sniffles, has an allergy attack, gets a stomach virus, or even has a bad day at work, the effects are seen in his sperm production. In fact, for many men sperm production can come to a temporary but complete halt simply due to a bad cold or flu.

Of course what gives sperm that sort of "indestructible" reputation is that a man's reproductive system has a powerful ability to regenerate itself and come back from even the most severe setbacks. Unlike your body, which could take a while to repair itself from a temporary fertility snafu, a man's body reacts much more quickly, and is capable of restoring the full power to sperm production within just 72 hours after problems clear.

That said, there are a few conditions and situations that can have a longer lasting, and sometimes – if not diagnosed and treated – even a permanent effect on his fertility.

To help insure that he takes care of any such problems straight away – before they cause any significant harm - I recommend that along with his yearly annual physical, he also ask his doctor about the three key fertility-related health problems explored in the next section.

Moreover, if he is experiencing any of the symptoms listed within this next section, encourage him to speak to his doctor right away. Doing so can not only save his fertility, but also help encourage a longer, happier, more fulfilling sex life, and in some instances, maybe even help save his life!

Problem # 1: Infections

In much the same way that infections – particularly STDs – can impact your fertility, so too can they affect your partner's fertility. Indeed, in many fertility centers around the world, undiagnosed reproductive infections in men is a leading cause of low sperm count, poor sperm motility and even defective sperm. And it is a leading cause of infertility in couples worldwide.

Among the infections most likely to impact male fertility include gonorrhea, syphilis, herpes, e-coli, HPV, as well as any number of bacterial infections. Male fertility can also be impacted by yeast infections, or urethral infections caused by bacteria in the urinary tract.

However, as is the case with women, the single most prominent cause of infection-related fertility problems in men is infection with the pathogen known as "Chlamydia." Why?

First, in up to 50% of all men who harbor this infection, there are no symptoms – so your partner might not even be aware that he is infected. Second this pathogen can be harbored in the body silently for many, many years – so it's very difficult to track down when and where it first occurred.

But while he may not have any outward symptoms, Chlamydia is silently working to destroy his ability to make healthy sperm. Chlamydia infections are also directly related to urethritis (male urinary tract infection), epididymitis (an infection of the tissues and organs directly involved in making sperm), epididymo-orchitis (an infection that ascends into the testicles) and prostatitis, an infection of the prostate gland. When left untreated, all of these infections can dramatically impact sperm production.

Moreover, there are also studies showing that a Chlamydia pathogen can actually attach directly on to sperm, affecting both motility and function. It also makes the disease extremely communicable, so if one partner has it, it's very likely the other does as well. As you just read, Chlamydia infection in women is also a leading cause of infertility.

Again the good news is that with a few simple tests your partner can be assured he has a clean bill of health. If an infection is detected , it normally requires only a short regimen of antibiotics and the infection clears. His fertility – and his sperm making ability – will be back to normal soon after.

While routine testing for infection – along with a sperm count and sperm culture – are important when a couple is having any problems getting pregnant, a man should be especially vigilant in seeking testing if he has any of the following symptoms in his genital region: Discoloration, growths, lesions, blisters, warts, abnormal penile discharge, as well as lumps, tenderness, swelling or rigidity of the testicles.

Problem # 2: Hormone Imbalance

Although we often associated the term "hormone imbalance" with women, the fact is, men can suffer from this problem as well. The three male fertility related hormones that can go out of balance include testosterone (the key hormone necessary for sperm production) as well as FSH and LH – which are the two brain hormones that direct the body to produce testosterone. So, it's easy to see how even a small decline in these hormones could have a major impact on his fertility.

While low FSH and LH don't really cause any overt symptoms he would recognize, if these hormones are under par chances are good that testosterone production is deficient as well (a condition known as "low T") – and here, he may see some symptoms. They can include loss of energy and fatigue, loss of muscle strength, weight gain, depression and loss of interest in things he enjoyed before. Perhaps most telling is a decreased sex drive - a man with low T can lose his desire for sex, or his sexual appetite may decreases from what it had been in the past.

Perhaps most telling is that a man with a low testosterone level will likely have a very low sperm count and without treatment to correct the deficiency could remain infertile.

Certainly, all men "slow down" a bit as they age. That said, if your partner is experiencing any of the above symptoms, and particularly if you are having problems getting pregnant, he must talk to his doctor about having a sperm count as well as being tested for testosterone and FSH. If these are low, then a test for LH may be necessary as well.

Should a problem be discovered, the only successful treatment is injections of the hormone HCG (human chorionic gonadatoprin), which works to reverse a low testosterone level, improve sperm count and restore fertility.

Problem # 3: Blood Sugar

One of the more significant health threats of our time is type II diabetes – and the precursor condition known as insulin resistance, both of which are a growing problem particularly among young men.

Besides increasing the risk of PCOS in women, blood sugar problems can also impact male fertility. In one study published recently in the journal *International Urology and Nephrology* doctors reported that men with type II diabetes were far more likely to suffer with infertility than men who did not have this disease.

Another study conducted in Belfast, Ireland and presented at the annual meeting of the European Society for Human Reproduction and Embryology reported that sperm samples taken from men with diabetes had a much higher rate of DNA damage than sperm taken from non-diabetic men.

Moreover, when left undiagnosed and untreated blood sugar problems eventually affect circulation in the tiny micro-vessels that line the penis. When these blood vessels undergo damage it can become very difficult for a man to have or maintain an erection – which in turn can make getting pregnant naturally almost impossible.

The good news: As you just read in the section on female fertility and insulin resistance, in most instances this condition, as well as adult-onset type II diabetes can quickly be controlled via simple changes in diet, and with regular exercise. When necessary, medications can help increase the body's sensitivity to insulin and in doing so help keep excess sugar out of the blood. And this, in turn can help keep sperm production humming along at a more normal rate. If a man has insulin-dependent diabetes, it's important to know he is still fertile and can still father a child, but it's vital that he be followed by a doctor and that sugar levels remain under control.

So, if you are having problems getting pregnant – and particularly if your partner is overweight - it's important that his blood sugar be tested. If a problem is found encourage him to work with his doctor to get and keep his sugar under good control. This is will not only improve his overall health and his fertility, but also help ensure that that his sexual potency and virility also remain intact for many years to come.

Eat, Love & Get Pregnant: A Few Final Words

It is my hope – as well as my belief – that most of you reading this book are young and healthy couples who, by making just a few small changes in your life and your lifestyle, will be pregnant before you know it! And in fact, statistics back up my beliefs.

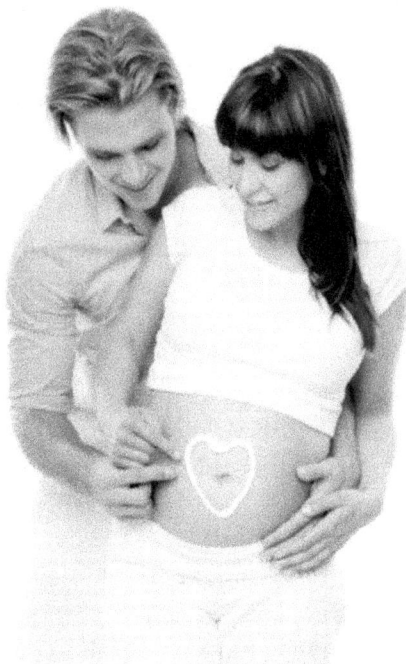

Indeed, for the overwhelming majority of couples under the age of 40, natural conception is not only possible, it's more than likely to occur. This is particularly true if you follow the outline in this book – which includes not just a good diet, good nutrition and a healthy fitness program, but also emphasizes the importance of love, compassion and understanding between you and your partner. It's a program that has been proven to work on thousands of couples – so I know it can work for you as well.

And while popular magazines, websites and newspapers are filled with headlines about infertility – and the high tech treatments necessary to get pregnant in the 21st century – you must keep this information in the proper perspective. The truth is, the actual percentage of couples who need medical help to get pregnant is still relatively small when viewed against the backdrop of the tens of millions of couples who conceive naturally.

At the same time, it would be unfair of me to suggest that none of you will ever need the help of your doctor or medical technologies to get pregnant - because that would not be true. Indeed, while all of the advice in this book can and will optimize your fertility in the best ways possible, still there are some couples for whom this won't be quite enough. This is why I will mention to you again that if you are under age 35 and not pregnant within 1 year of trying, or over 35 and not pregnant within six months, you should definitely consider having some baseline fertility tests to ensure that everything is okay.

And if in fact, if you do discover that you need some type of fertility treatment, it's important to remember that there are many options available to help you – far more than were available just a few short years ago.

Moreover, unlike in the past, today , in many states, insurance companies are bound by law to recognize infertility as a bona fide medical problem and as such they must pay for your treatments. This is something I fought long and hard for, for many years, and it is a topic that is very close to my heart. In fact, I am proud to say that I made many personal sacrifices and endured much criticism and hardship directed at me by the insurance companies because I continued to fight for the right of infertile couples to have their treatment covered. And while the fight is still not over – some states still will not recognize infertility as a problem - I am happy to say that by and large today many more insurance companies are now forced to pay for fertility treatments - because of the battles we continue to fight on your behalf.

In closing this chapter let me also remind you that there are myriad factors that can impact getting pregnant – and that most of these factors are under your control! Your diet, your nutritional status, your lifestyle, your stress levels – and most of all the relationship between you and your partner - are key factors that can all make a difference.

So, in this respect I strongly urge you to give the principals and guidelines in this book some time to work – and I urge you to have patience and most of all to relax. While it's important to keep positive thoughts in your mind about getting pregnant, it's also important that you do not become obsessive about the fear that you won't conceive.

Most important of all - continue to love, honor and nurture each other through this incredible journey you are taking together. Certainly, there will be times that are a bit stressful and difficult - particularly if you have been trying for a while now to conceive. Certainly, the road to happiness can be paved with a few sharp stones from time to time. But that said, if you continue to hold foremost in your mind the love you and your partner have for each, if you continue to work together, as a team, always as a team, I can promise that this journey you are on will be one of the most memorable in your life.

Most important, is to continue to talk to each, to listen to each other, and to honor each other's feelings through this entire process - and realize that a relationship is never 50-50. Sometimes you must give 75% while your partner is only able to give you 25% - but know in your heart that when you both give as much as you can, the team gets the entire 100% - and that is the winning formula upon which to build a strong family foundation.

Lastly, if you and your partner can learn to relax with the idea of becoming parents and give Mother Nature the room to work her baby-making magic, I can promise that you will become parents sooner than you realize.

Before I leave you for now, I'd like to remind you of these few words with which I started this book - the sentiments that I hope you and your partner will keep in your hearts:

- *To "Eat"* means to fill not just your tummy with nutritious foods, but to fill your heart and your soul with the positive emotions that make the world a better place to be.
- *To "Love"* means to not just love each other, but to love yourself, and to share your love freely & unconditionally with the new life you are about to create.
- *To "Get Pregnant"* means to not just conceive, but to fill your hearts and your life with the new found joy of creating a family, *your family* - the most important thing there is in life.

So my friends, Eat, Love, and Get Pregnant - and enjoy every blessed moment of it all!

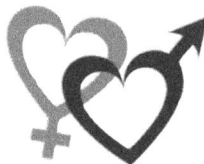

You can contact Dr. Lauersen any time, with any questions pertaining to pregnant or fertility by writing him direct at:
DrLauersen@NielsLauersenMD.org

Author Contact Information

NIELS LAUERSEN, M.D.,PH.D.

Web Address
www.NielsLauersenMD.org

Direct Email:
DrLauersen@NielsLauersenMD.org

COLETTE BOUCHEZ

Web Address:
www.ColetteBouchez.com

Direct Email:
ColetteBouchez@aol.com

Our Web Sites

www.GettingPregnantNow.org

www. GreenFertility.com

www.PamperingMom.com

www.EatLoveGetPregnant.com

www. FertilityDietGuide.com

www.ToGetPregnant.com

Our Blog: Fertility-Pregnancy.org

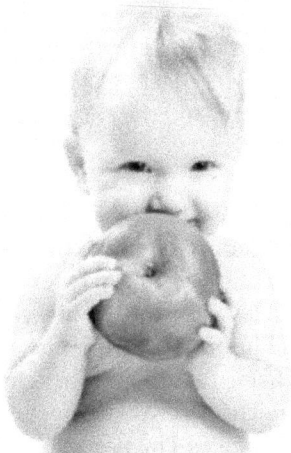

Join Us on Facebook at:
Facebook.com/FertilityNews

About Dr. Lauersen ...

In private practice for more than 30 years,
Dr. Niels Lauersen founded the New York Medical Center
for Reproductive Technology in 1984 to meet the growing
needs of the thousands of patients from the United States
and abroad who sought his expertise every year.

As a board certified obstetrician/gynecologist, as well as
a surgeon, Dr. Lauersen became world-renowned for his
expertise in the management of high risk pregnancy, the
treatment of endometriosis, PMS, & hormone imbalances
as well as the development of fertility - sparing surgeries to avoid hysterectomy.

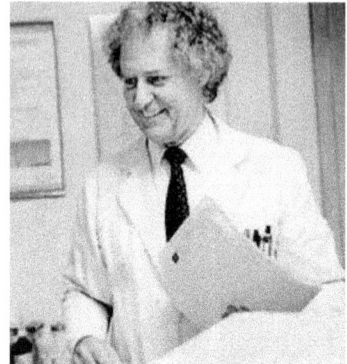

As a fertility expert, he was a founding member of the New York Society for Reproductive
Medicine and among the first private physicians in the New York area to offer a full range of
infertility treatments, including IVF, GIFT, and the newest ICSI, at his prestigious Park Avenue
fertility center.

Educated in his native Denmark, Dr. Lauersen received his American medical training at New
York Hospital-Cornell Medical Center, where he continued to do research and clinical patient
management and held a professorship in Obstetrics and Gynecology. His academic career
expanded, to include professorships at both the Mt. Sinai School of Medicine and New York
Medical College. In addition to his private practice, he was also on the clinical staff of Mt Sinai
Hospital, Lenox Hill Hospital, and St. Vincent's Medical Center, all in New York City.

During his active practice career, Dr. Lauersen was a Fellow of the American College of
Obstetricians and Gynecologists, and a member of the American Medical Association, the
Society For Gynecological Investigation, The American Fertility Society, and the NY Obstetrical
& Gynecological Society.

As the author of 14 books on women's health care, including the international best selling
fertility book *Getting Pregnant,* Dr. Lauersen has published more than 100 hundred scientific
medical papers, and wrote and edited several medical textbooks. He has lectured extensively
throughout the world and appeared on numerous national television and radio shows
including those hosted by Oprah Winfrey, Joan Hamburg, Regis Philbin, Phil Donahue, Sally
Jessy Raphael, Maury Povitch and Geraldo Rivera. He has been featured in articles in
newspapers and magazines worldwide including Time Magazine, The New York Times, New
York Magazine, The NY Daily News, People Magazine, The Los Angeles Times and others.

Currently, he is the medical director of GettingPregnantNow.org, one of the leading fertility
and pregnancy web sites as well as a principal in a medical publishing firm. He also a
consultant on the use of natural treatments in both men and women's health.

Dr. Lauersen also holds a European medical license for practice in the European Union.

About Colette Bouchez

As the author of 10 books on women's health and beauty , including an international best seller, and as founding editor of RedDressDiary.com, Colette Bouchez has become one of the most widely read journalists on the Internet. There are currently more than 100,000 pages of references to her work in major search engines, resulting in more than 1 million individual articles and book excerpts.

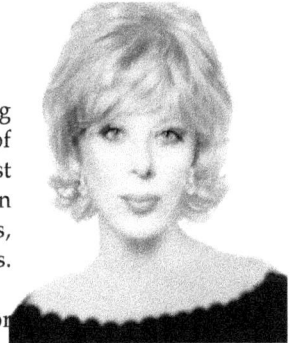

As the Editorial Director of ElleMediaNetwork, she is responsible for the editorial content and production of 14 web sites on health, beauty and style.

As the former content producer for WebMD's women's health, Ms. Bouchez was responsible for conceptualizing and creating content for some 35 million new and unique website readers every month.

Currently Ms. Bouchez is a health and beauty columnist for Examiner.com - National Edition where her weekly reports are seen by 22 million readers nationwide.

As a journalist Ms. Bouchez's work has been honored by many major medical organizations including: The American Cancer Society, The American Academy of Dermatology, The American College of Colon Surgeons, The Coalition of Breast Cancer Organizations, The Multiple Sclerosis Society, and Columbia School of Journalism for her health coverage following the aftermath of 9-11.

In 1996 she was the writer on the award winning WNBC TV team that produced a seven day report on breast cancer, taking the Emmy for best news documentary. In 1997 she was one of only a small number of journalists ever to be offered a fellowship at the University of Virginia College of Medicine.

In addition to her professional journalism memberships, in 2001 Ms. Bouchez became one of only a select few journalists to be admitted to the prestigious AMWA -American Medical Women's Association -the division of the AMA (American Medical Association) that honors female physicians and researchers.

Her reporting experience spans more than two decades and includes 14 years as senior medical reporter for the NY Daily News , founding member of the Health Day News Service and content producer for WebMD. She continues to be a contributing editor to major media including magazines published by the American College of Obstetricians & Gynecologists.

Experience also includes writing CME (continuing medical education) updates for the Excerpta Medica Publishing Group which helped prepare physicians for CME exams. Ms. Bouchez is also a medical/legal consultant for the prestigious law firm of Gerald Shargel and Associates where her medical research and data has often been used in the defense during numerous high profile murder trials

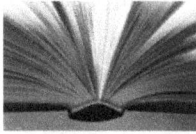

Other books
by Niels H. Lauersen, M.D., Ph.D.

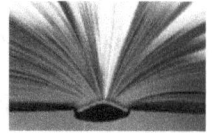

It's Your Body
Listen To Your Body
PMS & You
Childbirth With Love
The Endometriosis Answer Book
It's Your Pregnancy
Getting Pregnant
You're in Charge
The Breast Book
The New Fertility Diet Guide
Green Fertility
Eat, Love, Get Pregnant

Other books
by Colette Bouchez

Getting Pregnant
The V Zone
Is It Healthy - Is It Harmful?
Your Perfectly Pampered Pregnancy
Your Perfectly Pampered Menopause
The Hot Flash Solution
The New Fertility Diet Guide
Green Fertility
Eat, Love, Get Pregnant

**Visit IvyLeaguePress.com for more
information on purchasing any of these books.**

INDEX

___

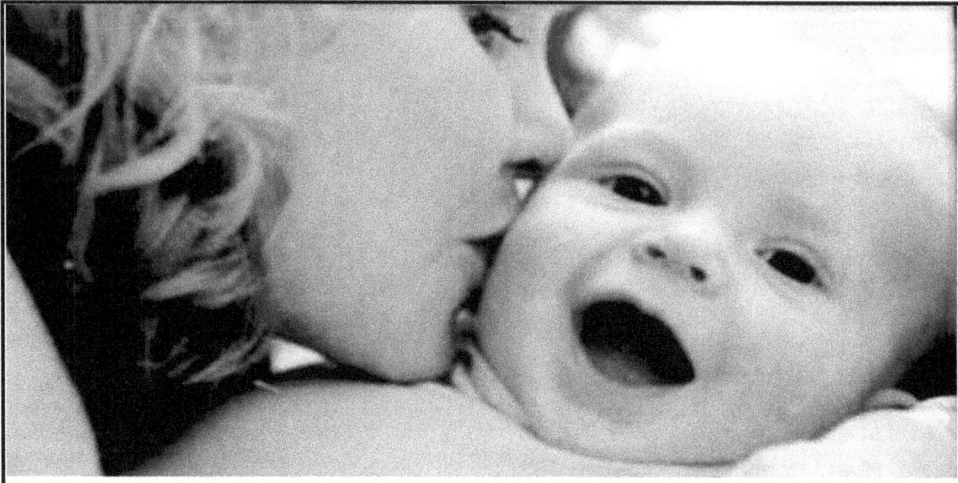

The Classic Best Seller -
Completely Revised & Updated

Getting Pregnant

WHAT YOU NEED TO KNOW RIGHT NOW!

BREAKTHROUGH TECHNIQUES FOR TREATING INFERTILITY PLUS:

* How To Get Pregnant Fast
* Six New Ways To Avoid Miscarriage
* The New IVF - How It Can Help You
* Gender Selection: What You Should Know
* New Treatments for Male Fertility
* 7 Super Fertility Threats & How To Avoid Them
* Your Fertility From 9 - 5
And So Much More!

By Niels H. Lauersen, M.D., Ph.D.
& Colette Bouchez

Getting Pregnant:
What You Need To Know Now!

From the authors of "Green Fertility " and " Eat, Love, Get Pregnant" comes a classic, best selling book on getting pregnant for over two decades! Now fully updated, discover why tens of thousands of couples already call this book their "Fertility Bible"!

VOTED # 1 By New Moms!

Getting Pregnant is the *only book* to combine the latest technologies with the best self -help advice to give you EVERY option for getting pregnant fast & easy!

From the best self-help fertility boosters to the most sophisticated medical fertility treatments you'll find all the information you need to make your pregnancy dreams come true!

Plus on our Website: Ask The Fertility Expert - Get a free personalized email answer to any question about getting pregnant direct to you from a fertility doctor!

So don't wait!
Pick up your copy of

Getting Pregnant

Available at Amazon.com, Barnes & Noble & fine bookstores nationwide.

And be sure to visit
GettingPregnantNow.org -
It's the website that will change your life!

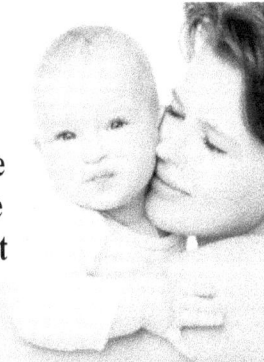

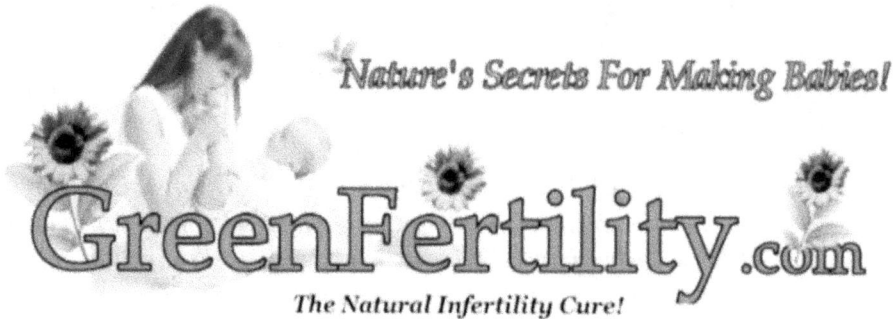

Nature's Secrets For Making Babies!

GreenFertility.com

The Natural Infertility Cure!

A revolutionary approach to getting pregnant
that pairs the power of *ancient holistic wisdom* with
new data on *medically proven natural treatments* to
offer couples a fast, easy, natural way to maximize their
fertility, get pregnant faster and have
a healthier baby!

By the authors of the best selling fertility book for over two decades comes this brand new book on how to boost fertility naturally, for a brand new generation of parents-to-be!

So whether you have been infertile and
unable to conceive for a while, or just
starting your fertility journey, Green
Fertility will help you get there - faster,
easier and naturally!

To learn more visit …

GreenFertility.com

*Or pick up a copy of **Green Fertility: Nature's Secrets for Making Babies**
available at Amazon.com, Barnes&Noble, & fine bookstores worldwide.*

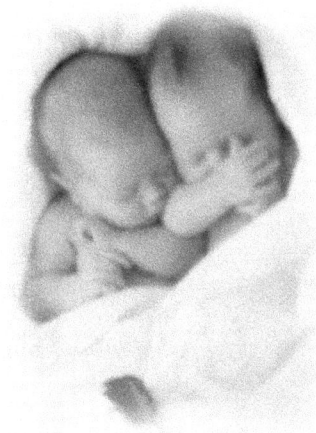

PamperingMom.com

- Health Advice
- Symptom Tracker
- Fashion Advice
- Skin Care
- Pregnancy Make Up
- Total Body Care
- Pregnancy 9 to 5

And so much more!

"It will change everything you ever thought about being pregnant!"

AHappyBelly.com

Fertility Jewelry & Accessories

Tap into the centuries old wisdom of natural gemstone
jewelry designed to help encourage fertility and foster
a healthy, happy pregnancy!
Lead-free · natural gemstones ·
healthy, gorgeous designs that will
become a lasting memento of your
pregnancy !

www.ingramcontent.com/pod-product-compliance
Lightning Source LLC
Chambersburg PA
CBHW080046280326
41934CB00014B/3235

* 9 7 8 6 1 5 5 0 8 8 6 3 *